Quick Look Nursing:
Fluid and Electrolytes

Quick Look Nursing

Fluid and Electrolytes

Mary Baumberger-Henry, DNSc, RN
Widener University
Chester, Pennsylvania

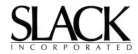

An innovative information, education, and management company
6900 Grove Road • Thorofare, NJ 08086

Printed in the United States of America.

Library of Congress Cataloging–in–Publication Data

Baumberger–Henry, Mary.
  Fluid and electrolytes / Mary Baumberger–Henry.
     p. ; cm. — (Quick look nursing)
  Includes bibliographical references and index.
  ISBN 1–55642–635–6 (alk. paper)
  1. Water–electrolyte imbalances—Nursing. 2. Body fluid disorders—Nursing. 3. Water–electrolyte balance (Physiology)
  [DNLM: 1. Water–Electrolyte Imbalance—Nurses' Instruction. WD 220 B347f 2004] I. Title. II. Series.
  RC630.B28 2004
  616.3'9920231—dc22
                              2004007932

Published by: SLACK Incorporated
                   6900 Grove Road
                   Thorofare, NJ 08086 USA
                   Telephone: 856–848–1000
                   Fax: 856–853–5991
                   www.slackbooks.com

   Last digit is print number: 10   9   8   7   6   5   4   3   2   1

Dedication

This book is dedicated to my husband, James Henry, and my brother–in–law, Tomas Henry, for all of their time, patience, and humor. They helped in more ways than they know.

Contents

About the Author

Mary Baumberger-Henry, DNSc, RN, is an assistant professor at Widener University in Chester, PA. She completed her Bachelor's of Science in Nursing at Mount Marty College, Yankton, SD. After 15 years of critical care nursing in medical/surgical, cardiac, and burn units, she received a Master's of Science in Critical Care and a Doctorate in Nursing Science from Widener University.

Preface

Fluid and Electrolytes is written for nursing students or students in allied health fields. It is written in a progressive style starting with the cellular membrane; advancing to tissues, organs, and systems; and finishing with the disease processes that affect the complete system. A physiological approach to the basic concepts of fluids and electrolytes and the need for acid/base balance in the body is used. Content includes disturbances of these properties and how the imbalance may affect the various systems of the body and consequent disease states.

Starting at the cellular level, Part I looks at the cell's membrane and how solutes are transported in and out of the cell. Part II involves the most important electrolytes in the body and how increased or decreased levels can influence body fluids and related clinical manifestations. Acid/base balance is the main content in Part III with a look at metabolic and respiratory control as well as interpretation of arterial blood gases. Part IV takes the reader beyond the cell with a look at organs and how four very important systems influence fluid, electrolyte, and acid/base balance. The book culminates with disease processes that stem from imbalances in the body. Written as a supplement for a text, *Fluid and Electrolytes* is a quick guide—from cell to system—that assists the reader in understanding a complex topic.

PART I
Basics

The Cell Membrane

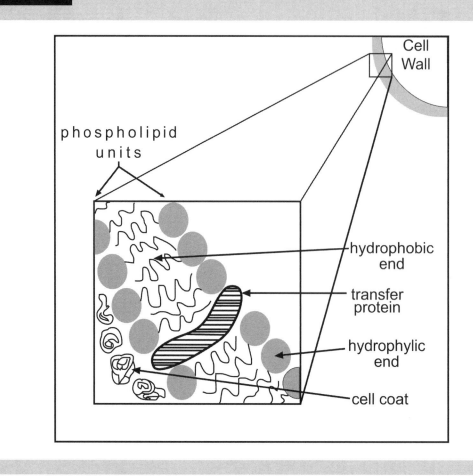

phospholipid units

Cell Wall

hydrophobic end

transfer protein

hydrophylic end

cell coat

Function

The smallest autonomous functional unit of the body is the cell. In its fetal form, it is undifferentiated. As growth continues, the cell differentiates into specific tissue types, forming organs and systems. The cell wall is a semipermeable membrane that separates the intracellular from the extracellular components, allowing for an exchange of materials through the membrane in the cell's effort to obtain energy, synthesize complex molecules, participate in electrical events, and replicate. The cell's ability to sense signals helps it respond to changes in its environment and adapt accordingly.

Composition

Phospholipids

The cell membrane is composed of phospholipids, fat–containing molecules of phosphate. These phospholipids are arranged with hydrophilic heads facing the outside of the membrane, which retains water and adheres to the neighboring cell. The tail end is hydrophobic and associates with other fatty groups to exclude the hydrophilic groups. Lipid composition determines the cell membrane's degree of fluidity. At a normal temperature, the composition resembles olive oil. As saturated lipids or cholesterol increase in content, the cell's membrane becomes less fluid.

Proteins

Protein molecules are the second major component of the cell membrane and the site where most of the functions of the cellular membrane occur. They transport lipid–insoluble particles, acting as carriers to pass these compounds directly through the membrane. Some proteins form ion channels for the exchange of electrolytes. The type of protein involved with a particular cell depends on that cell's function. The protein on a red blood cell (RBC), for example, has a particular flexible shape to allow the cell to thread its way through the small capillaries. In contrast, the protein of the renal tubular cell extends through the membrane in order to transport and exchange ions. Compounds such as glucose and nutrients are actively transported through the specific protein channels.

Cell Coat

Long chains of complex carbohydrates make up glycoproteins, glycolipids, and lectins that form the outside surface of the cell. This intricate coat helps in cell–to–cell recognition and adhesion. It contains antigens, which label the cell as self/nonself, or—as with RBCs—contains the ABO blood group antigens. If the cell coat becomes damaged or removed, the cell does have the capability to build a new coat, but it usually dies.

Active Transport

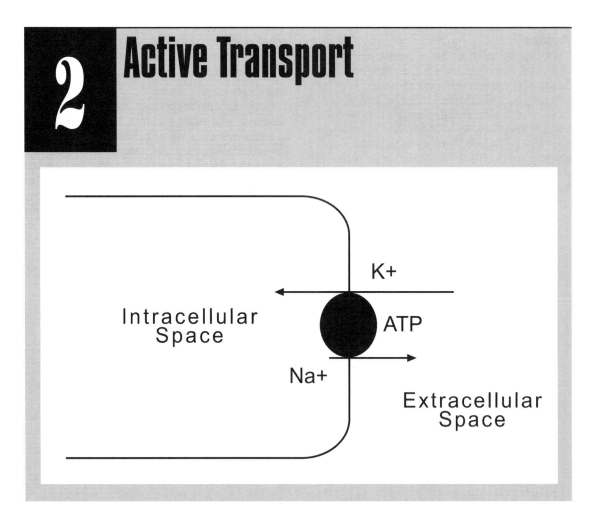

The cell is constantly at work, using energy and creating waste. Mechanisms are in place for the transport of substances across the cellular membrane; some are active and others are passive, such as diffusion, osmosis, and filtration. Active transport involves the use of energy to move molecules and is divided into primary and secondary active transport. Primary active transport uses the initial source of energy to carry the substance. Secondary active transport harnesses the energy obtained from the primary active transport and uses it as a cotransporter of a secondary substance.

Adenosine Triphosphate

Adenosine triphosphate (ATP) is a primary source of energy for moving compounds in and out of the cells. Molecules too large to pass through the cell's membrane, such as glucose, require an additional source of passive transport. ATP is the molecule containing high–energy phosphate bonds that is synthesized in the cell. ATP helps to carry a molecule against the con-

centration gradient (i.e., the difference in concentration between an area of greater solute concentration and an area of lesser solute concentration). This energy form cannot cross the plasma membrane to be stored; therefore, each cell is responsible for making its own ATP to meet its needs. Every cell has this capability, and the amount of energy needed is determined by that particular type of cell. High energy cardiac cells will require more ATP formation daily than cells with less demanding functions.

Sodium/Potassium Pump

One of the most efficient forms of active transport is the sodium/potassium pump. If sodium were allowed to accumulate inside the cell, water would follow, causing the cell to burst. Therefore, the sodium/potassium pump is present in all cells to keep potassium levels high and sodium levels low inside the cell and potassium levels low and sodium levels high outside the cell (see above figure). The high energy phosphate bond in ATP is split by the enzyme ATPase, releasing the energy needed to maintain the two electrolytes against the concentration gradient in their respective places. ATP is an important source of energy used by this pump to keep these vital gradients.

Secondary Transport

Secondary transport involves using the energy of a primary transport system to help transport another substance. Proteins with two binding sites help with this type of cotransportation. Frequently, sodium occupies one of the binding sites and is accompanied by another substance, such as glucose, which is too big to pass through the cell membrane. Amino acids are another substance that will occupy a site and cotransport with sodium.

3 Osmolality and Passive Transport

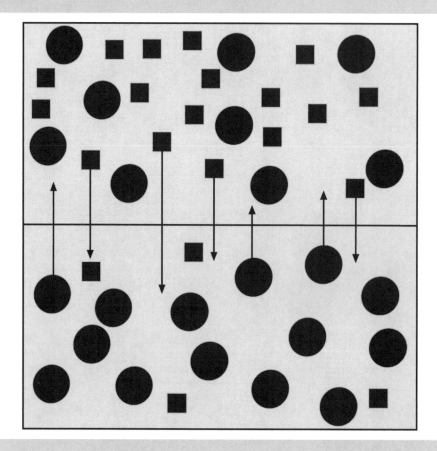

Frequently, the terms *osmolarity* (i.e., the osmolar concentration of 1 L of solution) and *osmolality* (i.e., the osmolar concentration in 1 kg of water) are used interchangeably. This switching of terms is accepted because 1 L of water is equal to 1 kg in weight. However, osmolarity is used most often when speaking of solutions/fluids outside the body and osmolality refers to fluids inside the body.

Whether ions are extracellular, such as sodium and chloride, or are primarily intracellular, such as potassium and phosphate, the equilibrium of fluids and electrolytes is controlled through active and passive transport. Passive transport is dependent on the osmolality of a solution involving movement from areas of greater to lesser concentration. A hyperosmolar

solution has a higher concentration of ions as compared to a hypo–osmolar solution. Osmosis and diffusion are two examples of passive transport.

Osmolality

The semipermeable membrane of the cell allows for a constant movement of some solutes while others remain confined within their boundaries. Whether confined or free to move, a solution's osmotic concentration is determined by the amount of dissolved particles. The normal range for serum osmolality is 280 to 295 milliosmoles per kilogram (mOsm/kg). Blood values that fall below this range indicate a hypo–osmolar state and those that are greater than 295 mOsm/kg are considered a hyperosmolar state.

The following formula is used to determine serum osmolality:

$$2 \times \text{serum Na} + \frac{\text{BUN}}{3} + \frac{\text{glucose}}{18} = \text{serum osmolality (mOsm/kg)}$$

However, sodium is the primary ion in the extracellular fluid (ECF) (range 136 to 148 mEq/L); therefore, simply doubling the serum sodium level will give one an estimate of the total plasma osmolality.

Passive Transport

Osmosis

Water is constantly shifting through the semipermeable membrane of the cell to the interstitial space or to the blood vessels and back in an effort to maintain a state of equilibrium. Unlike electrolytes, which require a special transport mechanism, water flows freely through the cell membrane, traveling between the intracellular and extracellular compartments using the passive movement of osmosis. Osmosis is the distribution of water from a lesser area of solute concentration to a higher area of solute concentration. The direction is determined by the concentration of particles on either side of the cell membrane. For example, when a state of intracellular hyperosmolarity exists, water shifts from the area of lower solute concentration and more fluid (i.e., the interstitial area) to the intracellular area with a higher solute concentration and less fluid. Osmosis stops when the concentration of solutes on both sides of the membrane becomes equalized.

Diffusion

Diffusion refers to the movement of solutes from a state of higher concentration to that of a lower concentration. Like osmosis, this is a passive movement that does not require energy. The rate of movement, however, is dependent on the availability of openings in the cell membrane, the total number of particles, and the kinetic movement of the particles. Increased temperatures affect diffusion. A higher temperature increases the thermal motion of the molecules, creating a greater diffusion process. Molecules will diffuse until there is an equal distribution on both sides of the membrane.

4 Fluid Compartments

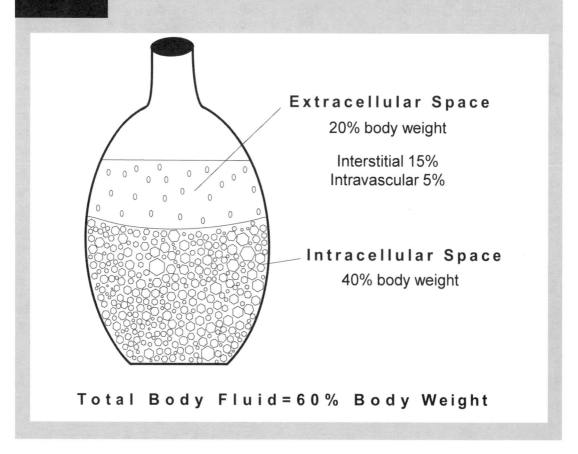

Extracellular Space
20% body weight

Interstitial 15%
Intravascular 5%

Intracellular Space
40% body weight

Total Body Fluid = 60% Body Weight

In the healthy individual, the fluid compartments maintain a constant environment through homeostasis. To stay within a narrow physiologic range, the body exchanges solutes and water between compartments, compensating for conditions that increase or decrease losses.

The body can be divided into two major fluid compartments: the intracellular and extracellular. The cell membrane serves as the initial barrier for substances to move to or from the intracellular compartment.

Intracellular Fluid

The intracellular fluid (ICF), or water within the billions of body cells, makes up approximately two–thirds of the body's water and 40% of body weight. The larger of the two compartments, the ICF is rich in the electrolytes, potassium, magnesium, inorganic and organic phosphates, as well as proteins.

Extracellular Fluid

The ECF compartment contains all the fluid outside the cell and is further divided into the interstitial, or fluid spaces between cells, and the intravascular, or blood vessel compartments. The interstitial fluid accounts for approximately 15% of body weight and the intravascular compartment contributes only 5% to the body weight of an average adult. The ECF is rich in the electrolytes sodium, chloride, and bicarbonate (HCO_3). When blood tests of serum electrolytes are drawn, it is the ECF that is measured for electrolyte levels, not the ICF.

Transcellular Fluid

A third compartment that will be mentioned briefly is the transcellular fluid compartment. This compartment includes fluid located in the peritoneal, pleural, and pericardial cavities as well as cerebrospinal fluid and fluid within the joint spaces and gastrointestinal (GI) tract. The transcellular space contributes approximately 1% of the body fluid, but this amount can increase when fluid collects in one of the compartments, such as the peritoneal cavity. If there is a significant increase in fluid within the transcellular space, it may be termed a *third space* since the fluid is not easily exchanged with the remaining ECF.

Total Body Water

Total body water (TBW) is made up of the fluids that exist in all the fluid compartments. This is approximately 60% of the body weight of an average adult. Expressed in kilograms, 1 L of fluid is the equivalent of 2.2 lb (1 kg). Because fat is hydrophobic, fat cells contain less water; therefore, an obese person will have less body water than a normal weight adult. In contrast to this, a newborn infant's weight is approximately 75% to 80% TBW. As we age, the body's water content decreases to approximately 45% due to the loss of skeletal muscle mass.

	Extracellular	Intracellular
C A T I O N S	Sodium 135-148mEq/L Potassium 3.5-5.3mEq/L Calcium 8.5-10.5mg/dl Magnesium 1.8-2.7mg/dl	Sodium 10-14mEq/L Potassium 140-150mEq/L Calcium <1mEq/L Magnesium 40mEq/kg
A N I O N S	Bicarbonate 23-27mEq/L Chloride 98-106mEq/L Phosphate 2.5-4.5mg/dl Proteins 16mEq/L Other anions 8mEq/L	Bicarbonate 7-10mEq/L Chloride 3-4mEq/L Phosphate 40-95 mEq/L Proteins 54mEq/L Other anions 31-86mEq/L

Values differ among laboratories
by patient nutritional status

Electrolytes are divided into positively and negatively charged groups called *cations* (+) and *anions* (–). Single or multiple charges denote their strength, or valence. Sodium and potassium are the predominant monovalent, single charge cations, while chloride represents a major monovalent anion. Calcium and magnesium represent divalent, double charge cations vital in many body functions. These electrolytes are measured in milliequivalents. Divalent ions have a stronger bond than monovalent ions. For example, two monovalent anions will attempt to maintain an electrochemical balance by combining with one divalent cation (e.g., $Ca^{++} + 2CL^- = CaCl_2$).

Unity of Charge

Within a single cell or the body as a whole, there must be a balance of electrical charges. Every exchange between spaces must conform to this electrical unity. If a positively charged molecule moves into a cell, another positively charged molecule must leave. Likewise, all cations must be balanced with appropriate anions within a body space or within a single cell.

Electrolyte Distribution

Electrolytes are distributed differently in the ECF and ICF compartments. In the ECF, sodium is the most abundant and powerful cation and chloride is the most abundant anion. Both sodium and chloride help maintain fluid volume in the body. Sodium is the manager of ECF osmolality. Any shift in sodium among the fluid compartments will affect fluid and solute ratios.

In the ICF compartment, potassium is the most abundant cation and phosphorus (phosphate) the most abundant anion. As an intracellular giant, potassium helps to control the osmolarity of the ICF and regulates the cell's electrical charge. If potassium is pulled from the cell, such as during acid/base imbalances, the electrical conductivity of the cell can change dramatically, resulting in a wide range of metabolic dysfunctions. Phosphorus, as the major intracellular anion, acts as a hydrogen buffer with acid/base balance. It is also vital for promoting energy storage.

Other cations, such as magnesium, have a larger concentration in the intracellular compartment, as compared to calcium, which maintains a fairly even balance between the intracellular and extracellular compartments. Both play a major role in enzymatic processes and electrical balance of the cell maintenance.

6 Acid/Base

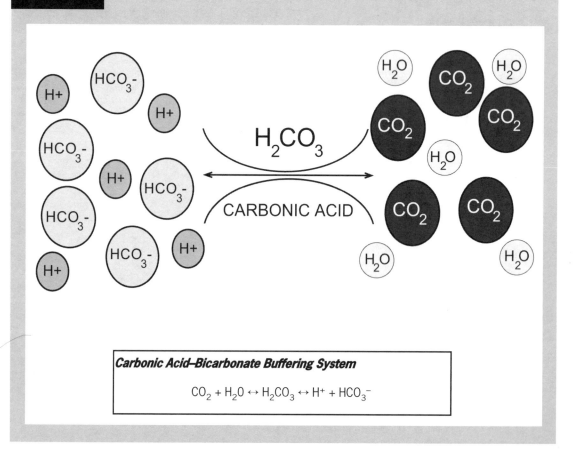

Carbonic Acid–Bicarbonate Buffering System

$$CO_2 + H_2O \leftrightarrow H_2CO_3 \leftrightarrow H^+ + HCO_3^-$$

The acid/base balance must be maintained in the body fluid. This balance can easily be upset by pathological conditions, such as infection; inappropriate use of medications; or trauma. At times, the acid/base imbalance itself can be more detrimental to the outcome of the patient's health than the initial cause of the person's illness.

The hydrogen ion (H^+) concentration in body fluids is very small, around 0.0000001 mg/L or 10^{-7}. Because the H^+ ion concentration is so low, the power of hydrogen (pH) is expressed as the negative logarithm, 10^{-7} with the neutral point of a pH of 7.0 in the clinical setting. The pH value is inversely related to the H^+ ion concentration; therefore, as the pH decreases, the solution becomes more concentrated with H^+ ions, and as the pH rises, the solution becomes less concentrated with H^+ ions. In the body, fluids with a pH <7.40 are considered to be acidic; those with a pH >7.40 are alkaline.

Acids are donors of the H^+ ion and form as end products of the metabolism of protein, fats, and carbohydrates. The body is constantly producing acids as end products of metabolism. Acids must be excreted to maintain a healthy metabolic balance. A base substance consists of molecules that accept the H^+ ion, helping to balance the acid content.

Three regulatory mechanisms (i.e., buffers, the respiratory system, and the renal system) maintain the short– and long–term acid/base status of the body. Of the three, buffers react immediately to an acid/base imbalance by absorbing the excessive acid and preventing abnormal changes in the pH. The respiratory system responds in minutes to an acid imbalance but has a limited capacity and takes hours to reach maximum effectiveness. The slowest of the regulatory mechanisms is the renal system, which takes from 2 to 3 days for a maximal response but has a greater potential to maintain the proper balance for a longer period of time.

Proteins and bicarbonate are two buffering systems that help control the pH of body fluids. Proteins, such as albumin, release or bind with the H^+ ion. Primarily located within the cell, proteins will bind with CO_2 or H^+ as the acid diffuses across the cell membrane. Buffering systems contain a weak acid and a base. The weak acid releases H^+ when the body becomes too alkaline and when the body becomes too acidic, the base binds with H^+. Carbonic acid (H_2CO_2) and bicarbonate (HCO_3) are the predominant buffers in the plasma and remain in a chemical equilibrium when homeostasis is maintained. When an acid/base imbalance occurs, however, they are available to assist the pH back to a normal value through the respiratory and/or the renal systems.

The respiratory system lowers acidity by increasing the respiratory rate and therefore, exhaling increased amounts of CO_2. The renal system has the ability to either conserve or generate new bicarbonate from CO_2 and H_2O. It regulates excess acid by secreting hydrogen into the urine as well as reabsorbing bicarbonate in the distal tubule. When CO_2 and H_2O form H_2CO_3, carbonic anhydrase catalyzes the reaction, forming H^+ and HCO_3. The H+ is buffered by phosphate or ammonia and excreted while bicarbonate is reabsorbed contributing to the alkalinity of the plasma (see p. 12).

7 Fluid Homeostasis

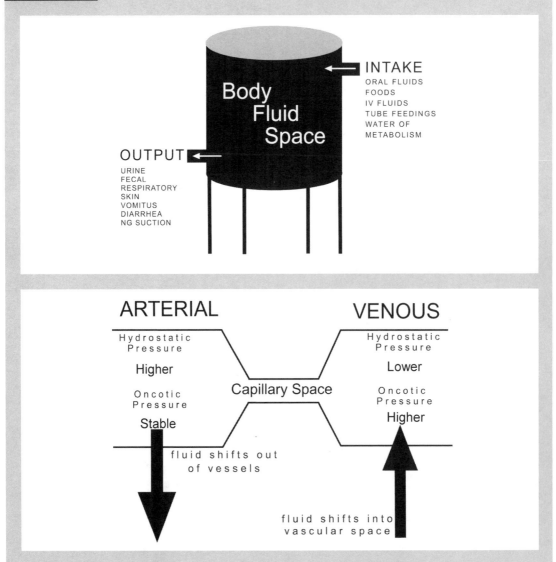

Fluid Homeostasis

Body fluid has multiple functions, including maintaining body temperature, transporting oxygen and chemicals, and eliminating wastes. Maintaining homeostasis of fluid in the various compartments of the body involves balancing fluid intake, fluid absorption, fluid distribution, and fluid excretion.

Fluid Intake

Normal fluid intake involves drinking fluids orally and ingesting fluids through food. Other methods of fluid intake include administration of water and liquid feedings through tubes inserted into the jejunum or gastric area. Intravenous (IV) fluids can be administered to those who need additional supplements to oral intake or those unable to ingest or absorb fluids via the

GI tract. The body also has the ability to generate its own water through metabolism or oxidation of nutrients, such as carbohydrates and fat.

Fluid Absorption

An increased osmolality will trigger the thirst center to initiate fluid intake. The fluid intake is then absorbed from the GI tract before reaching the vascular compartment. If fluid is administered through an IV, then it is directly instilled into the vascular compartment to help expand the extravascular or intravascular compartments.

Fluid Distribution

Once fluid has been absorbed into the vascular compartment, it is distributed between the vascular and interstitial compartments through filtration. Two forces control movement of fluid from the capillaries into the interstitial area: the capillary hydrostatic pressure and interstitial fluid osmotic (oncotic) pressure. Capillary hydrostatic pressure is vascular fluid pushing outward against the capillary walls, while the interstitial fluid osmotic (oncotic) pressure is the force supplied by the particles in the interstitial fluid that pull fluid into the interstitial area (see p. 14).

In addition, two forces—the capillary osmotic pressure and interstitial fluid hydrostatic pressure—move fluid from the interstitial fluid into the capillaries. They perform in the same manner as the pressures that pull fluid into the interstitial area except that the situation is reversed (i.e., fluid moves from the interstitial to the vascular area). Capillary osmotic (oncotic) pressure is the force of particles in the vascular fluid that pulls fluid into the capillary, and interstitial fluid hydrostatic pressure is the interstitial fluid pushing against the outside of the capillary walls. Since these forces are working against each other, the flow of fluid depends on the strongest opposing force.

The semipermeable cell membrane allows water to flow freely; therefore, fluid flows into the cell from the interstitial area by osmosis. Most electrolytes, however, require a transport system. The specific epithelial cells located in those particular areas restrict the flow of fluid found in the transcellular compartments.

Fluid Excretion

The most common areas of the body for fluid excretion are the bowels, skin, lungs, and kidneys. Fluid is lost through the bowels in fecal matter with increased loss during bouts of diarrhea. Sweat lost through the skin can be either profuse or the more natural occurrence of insensible loss. Fluid is lost through the lungs by exhalation, a normal and constant event. The largest amount of fluid loss, however, occurs through urine output. The essential urine output of the average individual is approximately 300 to 500 mL/day but averages approximately 1,500 mL/day.

Fluids can also be lost abnormally through emesis; fistulas and open, weeping wounds; or hemorrhage. Tubes used for drainage of body fluids, such as nasogastric suction, are another source of fluid loss. Normally, the body will compensate for such fluid losses; however, if the deficit exceeds intake, then a fluid imbalance will occur.

1. When a solution is more acidic, the pH value is _____ and when it has more base, the pH value is _____.

(A) Increased, decreased

(B) Increased, increased

(C) Decreased, increased

(D) Decreased, decreased

2. What are the two main fluid compartments of the body?

(A) Intracellular, extracellular

(B) Intracellular, interstitial

(C) Transcellular, extracellular

(D) Intracellular, intervascular

3. What is osmosis?

(A) Passive movement of solutes from a higher to a lower concentration

(B) A carrier that helps to transport glucose

(C) A movement activated by a thermal motion of molecules

(D) The movement of fluid from an area of low solute concentration to an area of higher solute concentration

4. What is a simple method for estimating plasma osmolarity?

(A) Add the BUN and glucose

(B) Double the serum sodium value

(C) Subtract the fasting glucose from the serum sodium

(D) Subtract the patient's potassium value from the serum sodium

5. Which molecule functions as a transport carrier system?

(A) Phospholipids

(B) Cholesterol

(C) Carbohydrates

(D) Protein

6. What is the regulatory mechanism that works the quickest in an acid/base imbalance?

(A) Buffering system

(B) Respiratory system

(C) Renal system

(D) Sympathetic nervous system (SNS)

7. Which of the following would be an abnormal way to take in fluid?

(A) Drinking fluids

(B) Ingesting foods

(C) Jejunostomy tube

(D) Eating apples

8. What is a substance that accepts the H^+ ion to balance the acid content?

(A) Base

(B) Acid

(C) Carbonic acid

(D) Protein

9. What is the most abundant cation in the ECF?

(A) Potassium

(B) Sodium

(C) Chloride

(D) Magnesium

10. What is the most abundant cation in the ICF?

(A) Potassium

(B) Sodium

(C) Chloride

(D) Magnesium

PART I: ANSWERS

1. The correct answer is C.

The pH value decreases with acidic solutions and increases with alkaline solutions. Body fluids that are more acidic have a pH less than 7.40 and fluids that are alkaline have a pH greater than 7.40.

2. The correct answer is A.

The body is composed of two major fluid compartments: the intracellular and extracellular. The extracellular compartment is further divided into the intravascular and interstitial.

3. The correct answer is D.

Osmosis is the passive movement of fluid from an area of high fluid and low solute to one of low fluid and high solute. Diffusion is the passive movement of solutes and can be activated by thermal motion. Protein is a carrier that helps to transport glucose.

4. The correct answer is B.

Doubling the sodium value is the easiest way to evaluate a patient's serum osmolality. A more complex formula exists to determine the absolute value.

5. The correct answer is D.

Protein molecules help in the transport of lipids and other molecules such as glucose.

6. The correct answer is A.

The quickest system for correcting acid/base imbalances is the buffering system. The respiratory system is also effective but may take hours to achieve maximum benefit. The renal system may take days to achieve maximum efficiency.

7. The correct answer is C.

An abnormal way to take in fluids is through any type of tube or IV line. Normal ingestion of fluid is by mouth through the intake of fluids or food.

8. The correct answer is A.

A base will readily accept the H^+ ion in an attempt to correct an imbalance. Acids are donators of the H^+ ion.

9. The correct answer is B.

Sodium is the most abundant cation in the ECF with a concentration of 135 to 145 mEq/L.

10. The correct answer is A.

Potassium is the most abundant cation in the ICF with a concentration of approximately 156 mEq/L.

PART II
Regulation of Fluids and Electrolytes

Water Balance

8

HYPOVOLEMIA   HYPEROSMOLALITY

THIRST

INCREASED ADH   ALDOSTERONE RELEASE

HOMEOSTASIS ACHIEVED

Regulating Water Levels

The healthy individual requires approximately 100 mL of water/100 calories ingested to help with metabolism and the elimination of wastes. The two main body mechanisms for regulating water levels are the thirst mechanism and antidiuretic hormone (ADH). Both methods are sensitive to osmolality as well as changes in ECF volume. Two hormones, aldosterone and atrial natriuretic peptide (ANP), are helpful in the elimination of sodium in the regulation of fluid overload.

Thirst

Thirst occurs when a loss of body water equals or exceeds 0.5% of the total body fluid. The perception of thirst, which occurs with even the smallest loss of fluid, is one of the best regulators of water balance. Depletion of the plasma volume, or hyperosmolality, is an event that activates the osmoreceptors in the hypothalamus, which triggers the sense of thirst.

Drinking fluids throughout the day is an unconscious event based on habit or social custom. One may feel thirsty when speaking for long periods of time, after consuming salty foods, or when breathing through the mouth. This dryness, however, is not truly associated with the body's hydration state. The sensation of thirst occurs when the osmoreceptors located near the thirst center of the hypothalamus are stimulated. This stimulation occurs due to cellular dehydration secondary to an increased extracellular osmolality or loss of blood. As one ages, the ability to sense thirst declines, a condition known as *hypodipsia*. This condition is particularly associated with those who have suffered a stroke and places this population at an increased risk for hyperosmolality and dehydration.

Antidiuretic Hormone

ADH is secreted by the posterior pituitary gland in response to stimulation from the hypothalamus when fluid osmolality increases secondary to a loss of water

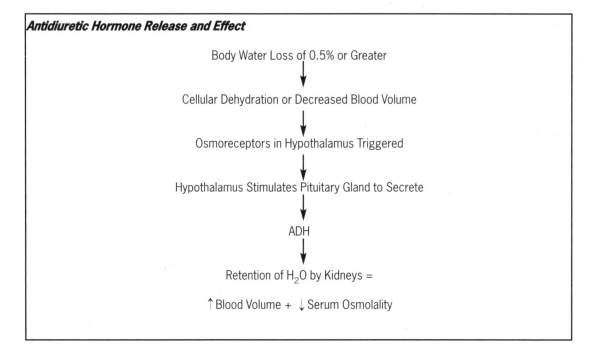

Antidiuretic Hormone Release and Effect

Body Water Loss of 0.5% or Greater

↓

Cellular Dehydration or Decreased Blood Volume

↓

Osmoreceptors in Hypothalamus Triggered

↓

Hypothalamus Stimulates Pituitary Gland to Secrete

↓

ADH

↓

Retention of H_2O by Kidneys =

↑ Blood Volume + ↓ Serum Osmolality

or excess sodium (i.e., hypernatremia). ADH is also secreted if the blood pressure decreases due to decreased blood volume. Fluid is pulled from the intracellular and interstitial areas into the intravascular compartment in an effort to increase the blood pressure. This decrease in fluid in the intracellular and interstitial compartments then stimulates the hypothalamic osmoreceptors.

The kidneys also play a fundamental role in fluid balance. When the thirst center is stimulated, ADH is released by the posterior pituitary to act on the distal and collecting tubules of the nephron, causing reabsorption of water into the plasma. Less water is excreted into the urine. As a result, urine concentration increases and plasma osmolality decreases and returns to normal (see Antidiuretic Hormone Release and Effect above).

The baroreceptors, which are located in the aorta, carotid arches, and pulmonary artery, along with receptors found in the thoracic vessels and atria, are also sensitive to volume. When dehydration secondary to vomiting, diarrhea, or situations of excessive sweating occurs, these receptors sense the low fluid volume, which triggers the release of ADH.

Aldosterone

Aldosterone, a mineralocorticoid, regulates sodium balance. The secretion of aldosterone is controlled by low blood volume. In addition, it is secreted by the adrenal cortex when sodium levels are low and potassium levels are elevated. Acting on the distal tubule of the kidney, aldosterone increases the reabsorption of sodium and excretion of potassium in the urine. Through the reabsorption of sodium, water is drawn back into the vascular system, thus maintaining fluid balance.

Atrial Natriuretic Peptide

ANP is a hormone released when the atria of the heart muscle are overly stretched. Sensing this fluid overload, ANP stimulates the renal system to vasodilate the efferent and afferent arterioles, helping to increase blood flow to the nephron and therefore increase the glomerular filtration rate (GFR). Under the influence of ANP, aldosterone secretion is suppressed and the distal and collecting tubules are inhibited from reabsorbing sodium. ADH secretion is also controlled, thus preventing retention of water via the kidneys.

Fluid Overload

9

EXCESS INTAKE	INADEQUATE OUTPUT
EXCESS IV FLUID	CHF
BLOOD/PLASMA USE	CIRRHOSIS
HYPERTONIC FLUIDS	NEPHROTIC SYNDROME
EXCESS DIETARY SODIUM	HYPERALDOSTERONISM
COLLOID USE	LOW DIETARY PROTIEN
WATER INTOXICATION	STEROID USE
REMOBILIZATION OF EDEMA	

Manifestations Related to Extracellular Fluid Overload

- Pitting peripheral edema
- Periorbital edema
- Shortness of breath
- Shift of interstitial fluid to plasma
- Bounding pulse and jugular venous distension
- Anasarca
- Rapid weight gain
- Moist crackles
- Tachycardia
- Hypertension

Causes of Extracellular Fluid Overload

- Increased dietary sodium intake
- Hypertonic fluid administration
    - $D_5 1/2$ normal saline solution
    - $D_5 .9$ normal saline solution
    - D10
    - 3% normal saline solution
- Diabetes insipidus
- Congestive heart failure
- Cirrhosis
- Renal failure
- Cushing's syndrome
- Hyperaldosteronism

Fluid overload can occur in both the extracellular and intracellular compartments. ECF overload occurs in either the intravascular compartment or in the interstitial area. ICF overload occurs inside the cell and is known as *water intoxication*.

Extracellular Fluid Overload

Edema is the common term associated with fluid overload found in the interstitial or lung tissue. When an overabundance of fluid occurs in the intravascular compartment, the condition is known as *hypervolemia*. The cause for overhydration may be associated with excess sodium.

Situations exist, however, in which sodium and water remain in equal proportions with each other. This type of fluid overload, known as *isotonic fluid volume excess*, results from a decreased elimination of sodium and water. Normally, the body will compensate and attempt to restore the fluid balance through the homeostatic mechanisms associated with ADH, ANP, or aldosterone. If these mechanisms malfunction due to diseases or failing organs, hypervolemia will develop. The extra volume of fluid will put an excessive strain on the left side of the heart that over time will cause the heart to fail, allowing blood to back up into the pulmonary system and causing pulmonary edema. In other areas of the body, dependent edema results first in the sacrum and lower extremities then it becomes generalized throughout the body, a condition known as anasarca (see p. 22).

Causes of Extracellular Fluid Overload

Fluid overload may result from excessive sodium intake through diet or administration of hypertonic fluids. Inadequate sodium or water elimination resulting in fluid overload may occur with conditions of hyperaldosteronism; Cushing's syndrome; and renal, liver, or congestive heart failure (CHF). A water deficit resulting from excessive diarrhea, diaphoresis, diabetes insipidus (DI), or decreased ADH may also result in a fluid imbalance (see p. 22).

Treatment of Extracellular Fluid Overload

Excess sodium and fluid are the primary causes of extracellular overload; therefore, restricting them is part of the treatment. Depending on other factors, additional methods of therapy might be used. If pulmonary edema is the problem, then measures to decrease it should also be implemented. In this case, maintaining a high Fowler's position with oxygen administration is necessary along with the use of loop diuretics and morphine sulfate. If CHF is the problem, diuretics, digoxin and other inotropic and cardiovascular drugs, a low sodium diet, and fluid restriction would be the treatment. Therefore, one must look at the overall picture to determine which treatment will be most effective.

Intracellular Fluid Overload

ICF overload is known as *water intoxication*. Hypotonic fluid from the intravascular space moves by osmosis to an area of higher solute concentration inside the cell. Cells run the risk of rupturing if they become too overloaded with fluid, and the cerebral cells are the most sensitive and first to react to excess fluid. One of the first signs of cerebral edema is headache, which may or may not be accompanied by irritability, confusion, or anxiety. Other symptoms that may be experienced include nausea and vomiting, thirst, muscle weakness or twitching, and dyspnea on exertion. If the condition persists, a patient with water intoxication will demonstrate an elevated blood pressure, decreased pulse rate, and increased respirations (see p. 23).

Causes of Intracellular Fluid Overload

ICF overload results from an increased intake of IV hypotonic solutions, such as 0.45% normal saline solution or D_5W. Dextrose in water, which is considered to be an isotonic solution, becomes hypotonic as the body rapidly absorbs the sugar content of the solution. Another means of developing ICF overload is through the electrolyte–rich GI tract. When too much water is ingested or instilled into the GI tract, electrolytes are lost. This may occur, for example, when excessive free water is administered through nasogastric and feeding tubes or with excessive ingestion of water from a compulsive condition known as *psychogenic polydipsia*. ICF overload may also result from renal dysfunction, resulting in a decreased excretion of water or excess ADH secretion known as the *syndrome of inappropriate antidiuretic hormone* (SIADH). This syndrome results in a large amount of water reabsorption by the kidneys (see p. 23).

Treatment of Intracellular Fluid Overload

Treatment for ICF overload is restriction of oral, enteral, and parenteral fluid intake until the serum sodium level returns to a normal value. In severe cases, a hypertonic solution of 3% normal saline may be used to help shift the water overload from the cell. Caution should be used with this highly hypertonic solution. It should always be placed on an IV pump or controller and administered at a slow rate so the body can compensate. Also, the potential for fluid to merely shift from one compartment to another may occur, causing ECF overload. In this situation, an osmotic diuretic should be added to the treatment.

10 Fluid Deficit

INADEQUATE REPLACEMENT	EXCESSIVE LOSSES

Poor oral intake
   CVA
   Dementia
   Neglect
 	
Inadequate IV fluids
   Poor IV access
	GI losses
	   Vomiting
	   Diarrhea
	   NG suction
	Renal
	   Nephrosis
	   Postobstructive
	Metabolic
	   Diabetes mellitus
	   Diabetes insipidus
	Skin
	   Burns
	   Open wounds
	Third spaces
	   Ascites
	   Effusions

DEHYDRATION
70 KG ADULT EXAMPLE

DEHYDRATION=1-3%   1-2 LITER DEFICIT
   NO CLINICAL SIGNS
   THIRST AS ONLY SYMPTOM

MODERATE DEHYDRATION=3-6% 2-4 LITER DEFICIT
   DRY MEMBRANES, POOR SKIN TURGOR,
   POSTURAL HYPOTENSION, OLIGURIA, MILD
   TACHYPNEA/TACHYCARDIA,
   HEMOCONCENTRATION

SEVERE DEHYDRATION=6-9%   4-7 LITER DEFICIT
   INCREASING SEVERITY OF ABOVE SIGNS
   HYPOTENSION WITH SHOCK, ANURIA,
   ALTERED MENTAL STATUS, ACIDOSIS

Fluid volume deficit is a TBW deficit that is associated with a loss of sodium accompanied by water. Iso–osmolar fluid volume deficit occurs when sodium and water are lost in equal amounts. Hyperosmolar fluid volume deficit occurs when more fluid is lost than sodium, resulting in a higher serum osmolality than normal (>295 mOsm/kg). Fluid deficit results in conditions known as *dehydration* and *hypovolemia*.

Dehydration and Hypovolemia

When serum sodium levels rise in the vascular system due to a fluid loss, osmosis will cause water molecules to shift from the cell into the blood vessel to maintain homeostasis. Normally, this restores the fluid volume. The problem occurs when fluid continues to shift from the cell, causing the cell to shrink or dehydrate. When less fluid is available to exchange among the compartments of the body, the circulating blood volume decreases, causing hypovolemia and hypotension. Patients may manifest signs and symptoms of an altered level of consciousness. This can progress to hypovolemic shock if the condition goes untreated and fluid is not replaced (see p. 26, Dehydration).

Causes of Fluid Volume Deficit

In addition to inadequate fluid intake, multiple causes can result in dehydration or hypovolemia. Prolonged vomiting or diarrhea, GI fistula, suctioning, or draining abscesses can result in a loss of electrolytes or fluid. Metabolic problems, such as DI, contribute to the brain failing to secrete ADH (see Chapter 8), resulting in excessive diuresis. The patient produces large amounts of dilute urine and is very thirsty, but a balance between intake and output cannot occur. Burns cause fluid to shift from the vascular to the interstitial tissues surrounding the burned area, resulting in hypovolemia. In severe cases, fluid is allowed to shift to the peritoneal space along with protein and electrolytes, causing a third–spacing fluid shift known as *ascites* and contributing to a decrease in the circulating volume. Fever and excessive sweating allow for an increased loss of sodium and water through the skin and respiratory system (see Causes of Fluid Volume Deficit above).

Treatment of Fluid Volume Deficit

Clinical management depends on the cause of the condition, but generally includes replacement of fluids based on the percentage of lost body weight along with treatment of the underlying problem. For example, fluid management of the burn patient is based on body weight and percentage of the burned area. Normal saline solution and lactated Ringer's solution are isotonic fluids given intravenously to expand the circulating volume. Solutions such as D_5W are not given as replacement fluid since the body will immediately absorb the glucose, resulting in the administration of a hypotonic solution.

11 Sodium

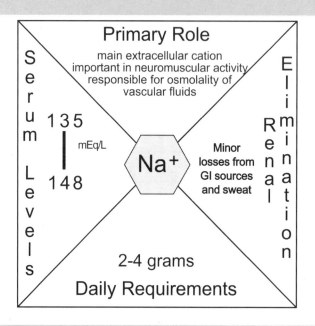

Primary Role

main extracellular cation
important in neuromuscular activity
responsible for osmolality of
vascular fluids

Serum Levels

Na⁺

135 | 148
mEq/L

Renal Elimination

Minor losses from GI sources and sweat

2-4 grams

Daily Requirements

RENIN-ANGIOTENSIN-ALDOSTERONE MECHANISM

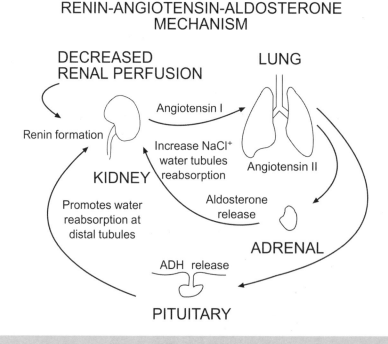

DECREASED RENAL PERFUSION

LUNG

Renin formation

Angiotensin I

KIDNEY

Increase NaCl⁺ water tubules reabsorption

Angiotensin II

Promotes water reabsorption at distal tubules

Aldosterone release

ADRENAL

ADH release

PITUITARY

Functions

Sodium is considered the most important cation in the ECF. Normal sodium levels in the extracellular compartment are 135 to 148 mEq/L compared to 10 to 14 mEq/L inside the cell. Sodium has several different functions. Primarily, it is responsible for the osmolality of the body's vascular fluids. Doubling the serum sodium will give one a rough estimate of the body's osmolality (see Chapter 3). It also has an affinity for chloride and helps maintain acid/base balance when combined with HCO_3.

The cellular membrane is impermeable to sodium, making the electrolyte dependent on the sodium/potassium pump for transportation in and out of the cell (see Chapter 2). Sodium is known for its ability to assist with the conduction of impulses along muscle and nerve fibers, and this is accomplished via the sodium/potassium pump. As sodium shifts into the cell, potassium shifts out, resulting in depolarization of the cell membrane. When sodium shifts back out of the cell, potassium shifts into the cell and the cell is considered repolarized. The sodium/potassium pump not only assists in maintaining fluid balance but also neuromuscular activity. Sodium plays a major role in maintaining homeostasis within the body. When serum sodium levels become elevated or below normal values, however, problems with fluid and acid/base balance as well as impulse conduction may occur.

Regulation of Sodium

Regulated by the kidneys and the hormone aldosterone, sodium's primary focus is control of serum osmolality levels and water retention. Its ability to attract fluid helps primarily with ECF distribution and control of vascular volume, which is highly important for tissue perfusion. When the vascular volume decreases, the kidney retains sodium in an effort to conserve fluid and, therefore, increase blood volume. The opposite occurs when the blood volume is increased (i.e., the kidney excretes sodium and water follows). The sympathetic nervous system (SNS) is responsible for the renal system's balance of sodium. The SNS modifies the GFR within the kidneys' nephrons in response to an increase or decrease in vascular volume. The higher the GFR, the more sodium that is excreted from the blood; when the GFR is decreased, more sodium is reabsorbed.

The renin–angiotensin–aldosterone mechanism also influences the amount of sodium that is secreted for maintenance of vascular volume and blood pressure. Renin is a small protein enzyme produced by the kidney and released in response to decreased renal blood flow. Renin then converts angiotensinogen, a circulating plasma protein, to angiotensin I. In turn, angiotensin I is converted to angiotensin II in the lungs, which initiates sodium reabsorption by the kidneys' tubules, and water follows to increase volume (see p. 28).

Aldosterone, a hormone secreted by the adrenal cortex, functions as part of a feedback loop that helps to conserve sodium. It acts on the renal tubules, stimulating them to hold onto water and sodium to normalize the sodium concentration and maintain fluid balance.

Maintaining Sodium Balance

The balance of sodium within the body can be maintained through a normal dietary intake of 2 to 4 g. One teaspoon of salt is the equivalent of 2.3 g of sodium; therefore, it is easy to see how supplements added to one's diet help in exceeding the normal intake to as much as 6 to 12 g/day. In addition to obvious sources of sodium, such as table salt and salty snack foods, hidden sources of sodium (see above) can quickly make up the normal daily intake. When dietary sodium is increased, however, the balance is not upset in the healthy person because the kidney will respond by excreting the excess intake.

Most sodium is lost through the kidney. Sodium can also be lost through the GI tract. Conditions that will increase the loss of sodium through the GI tract, however, must be excessive, such as prolonged vomiting/diarrhea, continuous GI suction, frequent tap water enemas, or the flushing of GI tubes with distilled water. Extensive burns can also result in the loss of sodium through the skin. Sweating may contribute to sodium loss through the skin; however, the loss is usually minimal unless a condition of excessive sweating exists, such as through strenuous and prolonged exercise.

12 Hypernatremia

```
H
Y
P
E
R                    Severe vomiting
N        RAPID       Hypertonic IV fluids
A        ONSET       Excessive sweating
T                    Poorly tolerated
R                    Correct rapidly
E
M
I                    CHF, renal failure
A                    Cushing's syndrome
         SLOW        Excessive salt intake
         ONSET       Poor water intake
                     Fluid shifts massive
                     Hypervolemia usual
                     Correct slowly
```

Causes of Hypernatremia

- Water loss
    - Diabetes insipidus
    - Watery diarrhea
    - Hypertonic tube feedings
    - Hyperventilation
    - Excessive sweating
    - Inability to drink water (e.g., un–conscious patient or confused elderly)

- Excessive sodium intake
    - Hypertonic intravenous solutions
        - $D_5$1/2 normal saline solution
        - D_5LR
        - D_5 normal saline solution
        - 3% normal saline solution

Causes

A serum sodium level of >148 mEq/L is considered hypernatremia. The osmolality in hypernatremia generally exceeds 295 mOsm/kg because it is an imbalance between the sodium and water levels in the body. Hypernatremia can be caused by either a greater loss of water compared to salt or an acute gain of salt compared to water (see above). If sodium levels are increased, water will flow via osmosis from inside and around the cell into the intravascular compartment. This causes intracellular and interstitial dehydration and may potentially lead to hypervolemia as fluid flows into the intravascular space.

Water Loss

A variety of situations exist that may result in an excessive loss of water from the body. Water may be lost from the body via urine as with DI (see Chapter 43) or with shifts between the ICF and ECF compartments

---
Manifestations of Hypernatremia

Skin

- Increased temperature, warm, flushed
- Dry mucous membranes
- Difficulty swallowing
- Increased thirst

Neurological

- Irritability
- Agitation
- Headache
- Seizures
- Coma

Cardiovascular

- Decreased blood pressure
- Tachycardia
- Weak, thready pulse

Renal

- Decreased urine output
---

during hemodialysis. The patient suffering from watery diarrhea may lose water from the GI tract. An increased intake of hypertonic tube feedings may lead to water loss with compartmental fluid shifts. The lungs lose water when a patient suffers from long–term tracheo-bronchitis or respiratory conditions causing hyperventilation.

Athletes have the potential to lose several liters of fluid during work out sessions in hot temperatures. When the body's set–point temperature is exceeded to extremes, however, heat cannot be dissipated by sweating or peripheral vasodilation and heat stroke results.

Problems may also arise when there is an inability to drink water or the situation involves an inactive thirst center. Hypernatremia makes one excessively thirsty; however, patients such as infants or those who are confused or unconscious cannot express this need.

Excessive Sodium Intake

Though an excessive intake of dietary sodium is an infrequent cause of hypernatremia, the condition may occur following therapeutic administration of hypertonic IV solutions containing sodium. Solutions that include sodium HCO_3 or 3% saline solutions may contribute to increased sodium levels. Corticosteroids may also cause hypernatremia.

Manifestations

Mild hypernatremia can essentially go unnoticed. As the situation increases in severity, however, water is lost and the sensation of thirst is triggered. The tongue feels rough and swallowing becomes difficult since the mucous membranes become dry and salivation decreases. The body temperature rises and the skin becomes warm and flushed. The renal system attempts to conserve fluids, resulting in decreased urine output. However, though the renal system is conserving fluid, the overall fluid volume in the body is low, causing a decrease in blood pressure that causes the heart to work harder and faster.

The most significant effect is evident in the central nervous system (CNS). When water is pulled from the cells of the CNS, dehydration of the brain and nerve cells occurs. The patient will initially demonstrate restlessness, irritability, and agitation. Complaints of headache may be present along with seizure activity. Eventually, reflexes decrease and coma results as the hypernatremia progresses (see above).

Treatment

Treatment depends on the cause and involves correcting the underlying condition. If the problem is related to a loss of water, treatment begins with replacement of the lost electrolytes and water. The use of oral glucose–electrolyte solutions is recommended for the less severe conditions. Salt–free solutions such as 5% dextrose and water can be administered intravenously if oral intake is compromised. Fluids should be replaced slowly because fluid will now shift to the intracellular compartment and cerebral edema could result if the shift occurs too rapidly. This is more likely to occur if the hypernatremic condition developed slowly or was chronic. Administering diuretics along with the IV fluids may also help to decrease sodium levels, but fluid balance must be carefully monitored.

13 Hyponatremia

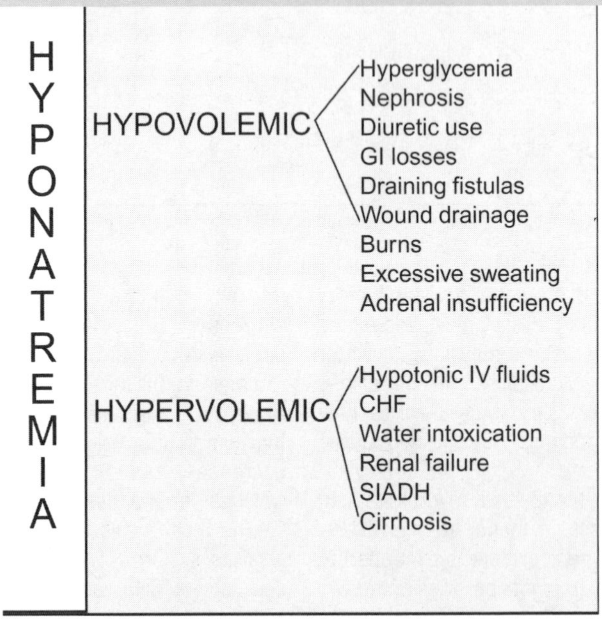

H
Y
P
O
N
A
T
R
E
M
I
A

HYPOVOLEMIC
- Hyperglycemia
- Nephrosis
- Diuretic use
- GI losses
- Draining fistulas
- Wound drainage
- Burns
- Excessive sweating
- Adrenal insufficiency

HYPERVOLEMIC
- Hypotonic IV fluids
- CHF
- Water intoxication
- Renal failure
- SIADH
- Cirrhosis

Causes of Hyponatremia

Hypovolemic Hyponatremia
- Vomiting
- Diarrhea
- Gastric suction
- Draining fistula
- Wound drainage
- Burns
- Excessive sweating
- Adrenal insufficiency

Hypo–osmolar/Hyperosmolar Hyponatremia
- Hyperglycemia

Hypervolemic Hyponatremia
- Hypotonic IV infusions
- Nephrotic syndrome
- CHF
- Cirrhosis

Manifestations of Hyponatremia

Neurological

- Headache
- Lethargy
- Personality change/confusion
- Absent/diminished reflexes
- Seizures
- Coma

Gastrointestinal

- Anorexia
- Impaired taste
- Abdominal cramps
- Nausea/vomiting
- Diarrhea

Hypovolemic Hyponatremia

- Poor skin turgor
- Dry cracked mucous membranes
- Orthostatic hypotension
- Rapid weak pulse
- Decreased hemodynamic values

Hypervolemic Hyponatremia

- Hypertension
- Rapid, bounding pulse
- Elevated hemodynamic values
- Pitting edema

Causes

Hyponatremia, or low serum sodium, results when the serum sodium falls below 135 mEq/L. The serum osmolality also becomes low, falling below 175 mOsm. In normal renal function, the body eliminates excess water by decreasing the release of ADH (see Chapter 8). When this homeostatic mechanism malfunctions, excess water is retained and fluid shifts occur. When more fluid than sodium is present in the intravascular compartment, fluid will shift via osmosis to the more concentrated area inside the cell.

Conditions resulting in an excessive sodium loss or excessive water gain lead to hyponatremia. It may also be caused by inadequate sodium intake, although this is atypical and is more likely to occur in patients who are on salt–restricted diets and who are also taking diuretics, such as the elderly (see p. 32).

Hypovolemic Hyponatremia

A dramatic decrease in ECF volume may lead to excessive sodium loss. This condition, also known as *hypovolemic hyponatremia*, may be caused by excessive loss of gastric secretions from vomiting, diarrhea, gastric suction, or fistulas (see p. 32). It may also occur in situations of excessive sweating, wound drainage, or burns. The sodium loss is not necessarily severe unless the fluid loss is replaced with excessive administration of hypotonic IV solutions or a large intake of water without electrolyte replacement, both of which produce a dilutional hyponatremia. If the problem is associated with the renal system, the cause may be due to adrenal insufficiency, resulting in a decreased reabsorption of sodium secondary to inadequate levels of aldosterone.

Hypervolemic Hyponatremia

Hypervolemic hyponatremia is the result of an increase in both water and sodium; however, the water gain is more significant. CHF, cirrhosis, overuse of hypotonic infusions, and nephrotic syndrome may be the cause of hypervolemic hyponatremia.

Hypo–Osmolar and Hyperosmolar Hyponatremia

Hyponatremia may also be described in relation to osmolality. When the TBW exceeds the normal level of sodium, a hypo–osmolar hyponatremia occurs. SIADH is an example of the body retaining too much water (see Chapter 43).

Hyperosmolar hyponatremia occurs with increased sugar levels (i.e., hyperglycemia). Glucose depends on insulin as a carrier system to cross the cell membrane. In a state of hyperglycemia, water shifts from the inside to the outside of the cell, an area of hyperosmolality caused by the increased glucose. Sodium, the major cation outside of the cell, then becomes diluted with the excess water, resulting in hyponatremia despite a condition of hyperosmolality.

Manifestations

The manifestations of hyponatremia are related to the fluid shift of water into the cell, resulting in an intracellular swelling and hypo–osmolality. The brain and nervous system are the most severely affected. The patient may manifest symptoms of headache, lethargy, and confusion that may lead to a more serious situation of seizures and coma if serum sodium levels are allowed to fall below 110 mEq/L. If the condition of hyponatremia develops slowly, signs and symptoms of the condition will not be manifested until the serum sodium level reaches 125 mEq/L. GI complaints of abdominal cramps, nausea, vomiting, and diarrhea may also be present.

Patients with hypovolemia will evidence poor skin turgor; dry, cracked mucous membranes; and orthostatic hypotension with a rapid weak pulse. Hemodynamic values may also be decreased. Patients with hyper–volemic hyponatremia, however, will show evidence of volume overload, such as hypertension; a rapid, bounding pulse; and elevated hemodynamic values. Pitting edema will also be present (see p. 33).

Treatment

As with any condition, alleviating the underlying cause is the first step toward treatment. If the cause is related to ADH, eliminating medications that may be contributing to the condition will help. Withholding or restricting fluid intake treats hypervolemic hyponatremia. IV fluids of normal saline solution may be given to patients with hypovolemic hyponatremia. If the serum sodium is less than 110 mEq/L, a hypertonic solution of 3% or 5% saline may be cautiously administered over a period of time along with loop diuretics to prevent fluid overload.

14 Potassium

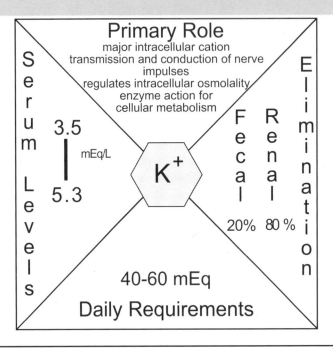

Primary Role
major intracellular cation
transmission and conduction of nerve impulses
regulates intracellular osmolality
enzyme action for cellular metabolism

Serum Levels
3.5
mEq/L
5.3

K^+

Fecal Renal
Elimination
20% 80%

40-60 mEq
Daily Requirements

Sources of Potassium

Dietary
- Fruits (e.g., oranges, bananas, cantaloupe, apricots)
- Dried fruits
- Vegetables (e.g., carrots, mushrooms, tomatoes, potatoes)
- Salt substitutes
- Nuts/seeds
- Chocolate
- Meats

Other
- IV fluids
- Potassium–penicillin
- Stored, transfused blood

Functions

Potassium is the primary intracellular cation, assuming the role of sodium inside the cells and regulating intracellular osmolality. Intracellular levels of potassium range from 140 to 150 mEq/L compared to the extracellular level of 3.5 to 5.3 mEq/L. The sodium/potassium active transport pump is responsible for maintaining this gradient. Primarily regulated by the renal system, 90% of potassium is routinely reabsorbed by the proximal tubule and loop of Henle, with the remainder selectively retained to maintain homeo–stasis. A normal dietary intake of 40 to 60 mEq will allow the average healthy person to balance these losses. Foods such as meats, vegetables, fresh and dried fruits, nuts, or chocolate are dietary sources (see p. 36).

With such a large intracellular stockpile, a small potassium transfer in or out of the cells will have a huge effect upon blood levels. Safe serum potassium levels have little room for variance. Renal dysfunction, medications, and tissue damage can quickly disrupt this delicate balance. Potassium's effect on maintaining the electrical potential of the cell membrane allows for the transmission of nerve impulses and muscle contraction of skeletal and cardiac muscle.

Regulation of Potassium

Potassium is primarily eliminated from the body through renal excretion. Nearly all potassium is filtered at the glomerulus with selective reabsorption occurring in the proximal tubule and loop of Henle. Variations in GFRs as well as hormonal influence determine how much potassium is to be retained. With intact renal function and sufficient free water, the body can adjust filtration rates to maintain homeostasis. When volume is required, sodium is reabsorbed to retain water through osmosis. An inverse relationship exists between sodium and potassium reabsorption in the distal tubules. Dehydration and acute blood loss lead to preferential reabsorption of sodium while leaving potassium in the urine filtrate. When renal function is impaired, excess amounts of potassium build as renal filtration rates decline. Hormonal influences through ADH and aldosterone further modulate reabsorption.

Maintaining Potassium Balance

Total body stores must be considered but are difficult to estimate from serum levels. Excessive losses may develop slowly through diuretic use or rapidly with profuse diarrhea depleting body stores. Measurement of these losses is difficult to document and must be anticipated clinically. Potassium shifts out of the cells to replace these losses. Such intracellular changes affect basic cellular functions, such as electric irritability of cardiac muscle. The reverse occurs with overload states as in renal insufficiency. Reduced excretion can easily drive serum levels beyond tolerance. Release of intracellular potassium from dying cells may be massive, as in the case of crush injuries to muscles or intravascular hemolysis from a transfusion reaction, increasing serum levels.

Shifts between body compartments are often more immediately critical. While diffusion pushes sodium into and potassium out of the cells, active transport pumps are constantly working to maintain the gradient. Any change in the cellular environment influences this delicate balance. Acidosis produces excess hydrogen cations that diffuse throughout all body compartments. As they shift intracellularly, potassium cations must shift out of the cells into the extracellular space to maintain electrical unity. Without altering total body stores, rapid changes in serum potassium levels can occur. Potassium also moves into cells with glucose during active transport. Using IV insulin can dangerously lower serum levels in ketoacidosis but can be lifesaving in the initial treatment of severe hyperkalemia.

15 Hyperkalemia

HYPERKALEMIA

IMPAIRED EXCRETION

ACUTE AND CHRONIC RENAL FAILURE
(decreased filtration)
ADDISON'S DISEASE
(decreased ADH production)
METABOLIC ACIDOSIS
(shift of H+/K+ from cells)

EXCESSIVE INTAKE

ORAL POTASSIUM SUPPLEMENTS

BLOOD TRANSFUSION

RAPID EXCESSIVE IV ADMINISTRATION

HYPERKALEMIC EFFECT ON ECG

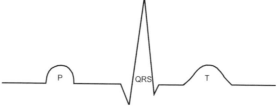

normal tracing (K+ levels between 3.5-5.3 mEq/L)

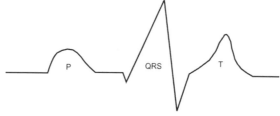

tall peaked T Wave, prolonged PR
interval, depressed ST segment,
QRS wider with K+ >7 mEq/L

Causes of Hyperkalemia

- Renal failure
- Multiple blood transfusions
- Medications (e.g., potassium–sparing diuretics, nonsteroidal anti–inflammatory drugs, angiotensin converting enzyme (ACE) inhibitors, digitalis, and potassium chloride via IV or by mouth [PO])
- Cellular injury
- Acidosis
- Diabetic ketoacidosis

Manifestations of Hyperkalemia

Neurological

- Vague muscle weakness
- Paresthesias
- Flaccid paralysis

Respiratory

- Respiratory depression from muscle weakness

Gastrointestinal

- Abdominal cramping
- Nausea
- Diarrhea

Cardiovascular

- Bradycardia
- Heart block
- Ventricular fibrillation
- Cardiac arrest

Causes

Potassium is the main intracellular ion. Hyperkalemia results when potassium accumulates in the ECF to a level greater than 5.5 mEq/L. Though the range for a normal potassium level is narrow (3.5 to 5.3 mEq/L), elevated potassium levels are unusual in the healthy person. Potassium becomes elevated in situations of decreased elimination, increased intake, multiple blood transfusions, or with a sudden shift of intracellular potassium to the extracellular compartment (see above).

The most common cause of hyperkalemia is decreased elimination secondary to renal failure. The renal system is primarily responsible for potassium excretion. When the kidneys are unable to respond to aldosterone (see Chapter 8), the ability to excrete potassium becomes diminished. Certain drugs such as potassium–sparing diuretics, nonsteroidal anti–inflammatory drugs, and angiotensin converting enzyme (ACE) inhibitors also work by inhibiting aldosterone and contributing to the retention of potassium. Elevated levels of digitalis inhibit the sodium/potassium pump, therefore inhibiting the balance of electrolytes the pump usually maintains.

Potassium levels can become elevated beyond the normal range with rapid IV administration of potassium chloride, particularly in the patient with compromised renal function. Lethal results occur when IV potassium is given directly without dilution. Potassium should never be given in this manner but always diluted with the recommended amount of an IV solution.

Cells that are crushed from injury or burns release intracellular potassium to the extracellular compartment. Potassium also moves from the ICF to the ECF during a state of acidosis as the H^+ ion is exchanged for the potassium ion or with a change in cell membrane permeability with situations causing hypoxia. Insulin is responsible for facilitating transportation of potassium into the cell; therefore, insulin deficits such as diabetes mellitus may also result in hyperkalemia.

Manifestations

The manifestations associated with an elevated potassium level sometimes involve the smooth muscle, which becomes hypopolarized. This affects the GI tract, initiating early symptoms of nausea, cramping, and diarrhea. A more common manifestation, however, is the effect on neuromuscular function. As the potassium level rises, the muscle cells become more hypopolarized so that the resting membrane potential lies above the threshold potential. This results in an inability of the cell to contract once it has discharged and the outcome is paresthesias, muscle weakness, and flaccid paralysis. The effect tends to start in the lower extremities, spreading to the trunk and eventually the respiratory muscles (see above).

The most serious effect of hyperkalemia, however, results in cardiac arrest. Dangerous dysrhythmias begin to develop when the serum potassium level reaches 7.0 mEq/L. Like the skeletal muscle, the cardiac muscle cells also become hypopolarized. The action potential and conduction velocity are decreased, resulting in dysrhythmias, some potentially lethal. The electrocardiogram evidences changes with the P wave, which is representative of atrial depolarization, becoming flattened. The PR interval becomes prolonged, indicating a delay between conduction of the atria to the ventricles. The QRS complex widens, representing a depressed depolarization of the ventricular muscle cell; the T segment becomes tall and peaked; and the ST segment becomes depressed, indicating a prolonged depolarization of the ventricular cardiac muscle (see p. 38).

The clinical manifestations may vary in individuals depending on the cause and rapidity of the elevation of potassium. Chronic conditions resulting in a slow increase in potassium levels allow the body to adjust and develop less severe side effects than a patient who experiences a sudden increase in potassium. Patients undergoing a rapid rise will more likely manifest the neuromuscular symptoms.

Treatment

Treatment depends on the cause and severity of the hyperkalemia. Patients with chronic renal failure (CRF) should be taught about the hidden dietary sources of potassium. In particular, certain salt substitutes contain large amounts of potassium and should be restricted in this client. If dialysis is an option, it will help to eliminate high potassium levels in acute as well as chronic conditions. In emergency situations, a combination of insulin and glucose may temporarily help to move potassium into the cell. Sodium polystyrene sulfonate, an exchange resin, combined with sorbitol absorbs potassium and may be given orally or rectally as a retention enema. Potassium is removed via the loose stool as it is replaced with sodium, which moves into the blood in exchange for potassium's movement into the intestine.

16 Hypokalemia

H Y P O K A L E M I A

EXCESSIVE LOSS

Diarrhea/vomiting
Fistula/suctioning
Diuresis after acute renal failure
Cushing's syndrome/steroid use

INADEQUATE INTAKE

Malnutrition
Alcoholism
Anorexia/restrictive diets
Inadequate IV replacement (i.e., TPN)

HYPOKALEMIC EFFECT ON ECG

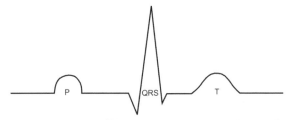

normal tracing (K+ levels between 3.5-5.3 mEq/L)

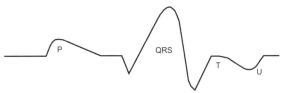

depressed ST segment, T wave
inversion, U waves (K+ level <3.5 mEq/L)

Causes of Hypokalemia	
• Improper diet (i.e., fad diets, potassium–deficient IV fluids)	• Steroids
	• CHF
• Medications (i.e., diuretics, laxatives)	• Liver diseases
• Gastrointestinal (i.e., suction, vomiting, diarrhea, fistulas)	• Nephritis
	• Cushing's syndrome
• Hyperaldosteronism	

Manifestations of Hypokalemia

Neuromuscular
- Bilateral extremity muscle weakness
- Paresthesias
- Hyporeflexia
- Leg cramps

Cardiovascular
- Weak irregular pulse
- Hypotension
- Electrocardiogram changes
- Lethal dysrhythmias
- Cardiac arrest

Gastrointestinal
- Diminished bowel function
- Abdominal distention
- Paralytic ileus
- Decreased bowel sounds
- Constipation

Renal
- Polyuria

Causes

A serum level of potassium below 3.5 mEq/L is considered hypokalemia. A low potassium level results from an inadequate intake, excessive loss, or a shift from the extracellular compartment to the intracellular compartment.

Decreased Intake

Insufficient potassium intake can occur from an improper diet. Fad diets or administration of large amounts of potassium–deficient IV fluids could result in hypokalemia (see above).

Excessive Loss

A large loss of potassium could occur with excessive use of diuretics. Potassium is lost via urine. Hypokalemia can result from overuse of diuretics, or use of diuretics that are too potent, without potassium supplementation. Intestinal fluids are also rich in potassium. Laxative abuse or loss of fluids through the GI system due to suction, vomiting, diarrhea, or fistulas can lead to a loss of potassium. Insulin (which shifts potassium into the cell), corticosteroids, and certain antibiotics can also be responsible for depleting potassium from the body.

Compartment Shifts

Conditions such as excessive gastric suctioning or vomiting can lead to alkalosis. During alkalosis, the H^+ ion exits the cell in exchange for the potassium ion, which enters the cell and causes an artificial loss of potassium. Other conditions, such as hyperaldosteronism, CHF, diseases of the liver, nephritis, and others, may lead to a hypokalemic state.

Manifestations

Hypokalemia is known for causing an altered function of skeletal and smooth muscle, allowing them to become hyperpolarized and less reactive to stimuli. A mild case of hypokalemia may start as bilateral muscle weakness, starting in the lower extremities with leg cramps and paresthesia, but if the potassium loss progresses, flaccid paralysis may occur. The complications ascend up the body, affecting the smooth muscle. The GI system may be affected with diminished bowel function, resulting in abdominal distention and possible paralytic ileus (see above). An extreme complication of respiratory paralysis may occur but happens infrequently.

The cardiac muscle cells initially become hyperpolarized with decreased potassium levels. As the levels become dangerously low, the cells become hypopolarized, resulting in an increased diastolic depolarization. This results in excitability of the cells and the development of ectopic beats. Decreased conduction velocity of impulses through the atrioventricular node and prolonging of the cardiac action potential occur. Such effects on the heart present as a weak and irregular pulse along with orthostatic hypotension. The electrocardiogram (ECG) may show a depressed ST segment, flattened T wave, and a U wave. The ectopic beats that irritate the ventricle may potentiate lethal dysrhythmias and eventual cardiac arrest. Hypokalemia especially affects the patient on digitalis glycosides, increasing the risk for digitalis toxicity (see p. 42).

Treatment

Treatment involves replacing the lost potassium. Monitoring serum laboratory values will determine the severity of the condition. If the situation is a mild loss of potassium, oral supplements may help raise the level. If the loss is more severe, IV potassium administration may be necessary. IV potassium is always diluted with IV solutions according to guidelines for recommended concentrations. It is never given undiluted IV push or bolus; administering potassium in this manner will result in cardiac arrest.

17 Calcium

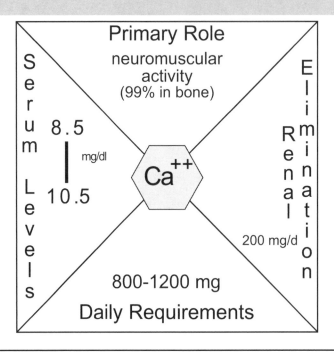

Primary Role

neuromuscular activity

(99% in bone)

Serum Levels

8.5 | mg/dl

10.5

Ca^{++}

Renal Elimination

200 mg/d

800-1200 mg

Daily Requirements

Calcium Food Sources
- Milk, yogurt, cheese, ice cream, tofu
- Canned salmon, sardines
- Broccoli, turnip greens, bok choy, kale
- Rhubarb
- Pinto beans
- Almonds
- Figs

Function

The normal range for total serum calcium is 8.5 to 10.5 mg/dL or 4.5 to 5.5 mEq/L. Ninety–nine percent of calcium is located in the bones and teeth and is responsible for the formation and firm structure of these body parts. This leaves 1% of calcium in the cells and fluid compartments, with the majority of that 1% in the extracellular compartment. Forty–one percent of this extracellular calcium is bound to the protein albu-

min. Therefore, when albumin levels decline, so does the calcium level. A small percentage is bound to citrate and other small organic ions. The remainder of calcium is ionized (unbound). The normal value for ionized calcium is 4.5 to 5.1 mg/dL or 2.2 to 2.5 mEq/L. This ionized or free calcium conducts the physiological functions, and any imbalances in the levels of ionized calcium result in hypocalcemia or hypercalcemia. Calcium functions in cellular permeability and in the contraction of cardiac, smooth, and skeletal muscle. It also plays a role in the blood–clotting process.

Regulation of Calcium

Calcium is ingested through food sources, especially dairy products and green leafy vegetables (see p. 46), and absorbed from the small intestine. Elimination occurs in the urine and feces. The minimum daily requirement is 800 to 1200 mg/day. This amount varies, however, with pregnancy, childhood, and conditions of osteoporosis. When calcium levels are low, the parathyroid hormone helps to regulate calcium by mobilizing it, pulling it out of the bones, and releasing it into the blood stream. This hormone also dictates kidney reabsorption and, along with vitamin D, promotes intestinal absorption of calcium in an effort to maintain regulation. In contrast to the parathyroid hormone, calcitonin—which is secreted by the thyroid gland—regulates elevated calcium levels by increasing calcium deposits in the bone, decreasing GI absorption, and increasing renal elimination of calcium.

Maintaining Calcium Balance

The extracellular levels of calcium are kept in balance in the healthy individual through dietary intake and reabsorption from bone and kidney. Vitamin D is essential for absorption of calcium from the available sources. An increased intake of calcium will not raise blood levels or be properly absorbed without vitamin D, which is easily obtained through sunshine and food sources such as dairy products.

18 Hypercalcemia

<table>
<tr><td rowspan="2" style="writing-mode: vertical-rl">HYPERCALCEMIA</td><td>

HIGH INTAKE or RELEASE

Calcium antacids
Calcium supplements
Bone destruction (tumor/immobilization)
Ectopic parathyroid hormone
Steroid therapy
Vitamin D
</td></tr>
<tr><td>

INADEQUATE OUTPUT

Renal failure
Thiazide diuretics
Increased parathyroid hormone
</td></tr>
</table>

Causes of Hypercalcemia

- Hyperparathyroidism
- Hypophosphatemia
- Cancer (i.e., lung, breast, ovary, prostate, GI, leukemia)
- Prolonged immobilization
- Multiple fractures
- Medications (i.e., thiazide diuretics, steroids, calcium supplements/antacids, vitamin D)

Causes

Hypercalcemia results when the movement of calcium into the circulation overwhelms the ability of the regulatory hormones or the renal system to eliminate excess calcium ions. Hypercalcemia is documented when the serum calcium level rises above 10.5 mg/dL or 5.5 mEq/L. Ionized serum calcium levels must rise above 5.25 mg/dL or 2.5 mEq/L for hypercalcemia to exist.

Hyperparathyroidism can be responsible for hypercalcemia due to the increased production of parathyroid hormone, which helps activate calcium from bone. A second cause for hypercalcemia is the destruction of bone secondary to malignant cells of certain cancers such as lung, breast, ovary, prostate, GI, and leukemia.

Less common causes of hypercalcemia are prolonged immobility or multiple fractures, leading to demineralization and the release of calcium from bone. Excessive vitamin D– or calcium–containing supplements can lead to increased intestinal absorption of calcium. A decreased excretion of calcium by the kid-

Manifestations of Hypercalcemia	
Cardiac	**Gastrointestinal**
• Ventricular dysrhythmias	• Anorexia
• Bradyarrhythmias	• Nausea/vomiting
• Heart block	• Constipation
• Asystole	• Pancreatitis
Neural	**Renal**
• Personality changes, psychosis, confusion	• Calculi
• Decreased memory	
• Stupor, possible coma	
• Lethargy, muscle weakness	
• Depressed reflexes	

neys through the use of thiazide diuretics can result in hypercalcemia. They are also known for promoting the action of parathyroid hormone helping to increase calcium reabsorption. Phosphorus is known to inhibit calcium absorption in the intestines; therefore, hypo–phosphatemia is related to hypercalcemia. The serum pH also has an inverse relationship with ionized calcium. As the pH level drops, resulting in acidosis, less calcium binds to protein, causing an increased ionized calcium level (see p. 48).

Manifestations

Calcium functions in the contraction of cardiac, skeletal, and smooth muscle, and hypercalcemia causes a decrease in cell membrane excitability. The heart muscle may respond through increased contractility demonstrated on the ECG as a shortened QT interval and decreased or diminished ST segment. Ventricular dysrhythmias, bradyarrhythmias, and heart block may develop into asystole. If the patient is taking digitalis, the responses to these conditions may be accentuated (see above).

Neural excitability decreases with hypercalcemia, allowing for a change in personality or a dulling of consciousness, stupor, and possible coma in more severe cases. Patients may complain of fatigue and muscle weakness. Muscle tone becomes decreased, and a hyporeflexia develops.

As a result of the smooth muscle being affected, GI symptoms of anorexia, nausea, vomiting, and constipation develop. Stones may develop, causing a blocking of the pancreatic ducts that results in pancreatitis.

The renal system is responsible for concentrating urine; however, in situations involving hypercalcemia, the high levels of calcium interfere with the action of ADH, causing diuresis and subsequent dehydration. Another problem resulting from elevated calcium levels is renal calculi.

Hypercalcemic crisis is the result of an acute situation generally stemming from malignant disease or hyperparathyroidism. This condition results in polyuria, which contributes to a state of dehydration, excessive thirst, fever, azotemia (i.e., a collection of nitrogenous waste products), an altered level of consciousness, and cardiac arrest. This rapid chain of events usually results in a high mortality rate.

Treatment

Treatment for hypercalcemia includes treating the underlying problem, keeping calcium from leaving bone, and allowing for renal excretion. Sodium and calcium are eliminated together; therefore, the combination of a normal saline solution and calcitonin can be rapidly administered followed by a loop diuretic such as furosemide. This will help with rapid diuresis of calcium. Rehydration is also important and must be closely monitored when diuresis is part of the treatment.

Drugs that inhibit bone reabsorption through inhibition of osteoclastic activity are the bisphosphonates and calcitonin. Plicamycin (mithramycin) and cortico–steroids help to inhibit bone reabsorption for cancer patients. Plicamycin is nephrotoxic and hepatotoxic, so it should be used with caution for long–term patients.

19 Hypocalcemia

H Y P O C A L C E M I A	**INADEQUATE INTAKE** VITAMIN DEFICIENCY POOR DIETARY CALCIUM SOURCES ALCOHOLISM LIMITS ABSORPTION (MEDICATIONS / CHRONIC DIARRHEA)
	EXCESSIVE LOSSES PRIMARY/SECONDARY HYPOPARATHYROIDISM RENAL FAILURE AND/OR HIGH PHOSPHATE ALKALOSIS (INCREASES PROTEIN BINDING) PANCREATITIS LAXATIVES

Causes of Hypocalcemia
- Alcoholism
- Pancreatitis
- GI problems (i.e., prolonged diarrhea, overuse of laxatives)
- CRF
- Decreased parathyroid hormone
- Hypoalbuminemia
- Hyperphosphatemia
- Medications (i.e., mithramycin, calcitonin, diuretics, cisplatin, gentamicin)

Causes

Hypocalcemia occurs when the calcium level falls below 8.5 mg/dL or 4.5 mEq/L. Hypocalcemic states occur through excessive loss of calcium from the body, a lack of ingestion, or absorption of the mineral. Alcoholics are particularly prone to developing hypo–calcemia secondary to a lack of intake and poor absorption related to a malnourished state. Pancreati- tis can result in hypocalcemia due to a decreased absorption and an increased excretion of calcium. Pancreatitis results in a decrease in pancreatic lipase, which normally helps with the digestion of dietary fats. Because the fats cannot be absorbed, calcium from the diet and then secreted into the intestine cannot be absorbed. Instead, calcium is bound to the undigested fat and excreted from the body.

Malabsorption of calcium occurs when the ion cannot be absorbed properly in the GI tract. Situations of prolonged diarrhea, overuse of laxatives, or increased intestinal motility will result in malabsorption. Calcium needs vitamin D for proper absorption. When certain medications interfere with vitamin D metabolism, such as anticonvulsants, calcium absorption suffers. CRF can also be the cause of poor absorption of calcium as the kidneys lose the ability to activate vitamin D.

Parathyroid hormone, which is responsible for kidney reabsorption and intestinal absorption of calcium, can be the cause of hypocalcemia if the parathyroid gland is removed. Thyroid surgery, hypomagnesemia, hypoparathyroidism, and tumors of or injury to the parathyroid gland can all result in reduced or a complete lack of parathyroid hormone.

Drugs known for decreased calcium reabsorption from bone are mithramycin and calcitonin. Diuretics, particularly the loop diuretics such as furosemide or ethacrynic acid, can bring about hypocalcemia by eliminating the ion through an increased urine output. Phosphates or drugs that lower serum magnesium, such as cisplatin or gentamicin, can also contribute to a low calcium level.

Because 41% of calcium binds to protein, calcium levels will also drop when protein (albumin) stores are low (i.e., hypoalbuminemia). Another cause of hypocalcemia is high phosphorus levels (see p. 50)

Manifestations

Calcium is important for determining the speed of ion fluxes causing muscle contraction; therefore, as hypercalcemia causes decreased muscle contraction and excitability, hypocalcemia causes increased muscle contraction and excitability. Action potentials of the muscle cell are easily generated with hypocalcemia. This excitability increases to the point of neuromuscular irritability manifested by a positive Trousseau's or Chvostek's sign, muscle twitching, paresthesias, and cramping, leading to potential tetany. Hyperactive reflexes may develop along with seizures. Cardiac dysrhythmias result from a prolonged plateau phase of the cardiac action potential. This affects atrioventricular and intraventricular conduction as well as myocardial contractility (see above).

Trousseau's and Chvostek's Signs

To test for a positive Trousseau's sign, occlude arterial blood flow to the hand for approximately 3 minutes. If this is followed by a carpopedal spasm (i.e., flexed wrist and metacarpophalangeal joints, extended interphalangeal joints, and adducted thumb), the test is positive for increased neuromuscular irritability. Tapping the facial nerve in front of the ear may produce a spasm of muscles in the cheek. This is indicative of a positive Chvostek's sign. Though these tests are reflective of increased neuromuscular irritability that may relate to hypocalcemia, they also may point to other conditions and should be interpreted with caution.

Treatment

Treatment depends on the underlying cause and treating the primary source of the problem. If the situation is acute, IV calcium gluconate or calcium chloride may be given. Vitamin D may be given to help absorption of oral calcium supplements in the GI tract if the condition becomes chronic.

20 Chloride

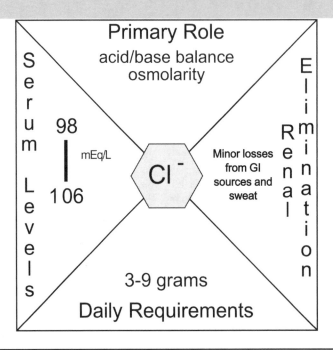

Primary Role
acid/base balance
osmolarity

Serum Levels

98 | mEq/L | 106

Cl⁻

Minor losses from GI sources and sweat

Renal Elimination

3-9 grams
Daily Requirements

Dietary Sources of Chloride
- Table salt
- Fruits (i.e., dates, bananas)
- Vegetables (i.e., spinach, celery)
- Fish
- Dairy products (i.e., cheese, milk, eggs)
- Processed meats and foods
- Soy sauce

Function

Serum chloride levels range between 98 to 106 mEq/L in the ECF and approximately 4 mEq/L in the ICF. Chloride, the most abundant anion in the ECF, can be found in gastric secretions, pancreatic juices, and bile. It is most plentiful in the cerebrospinal fluid where it joins with sodium. Its negative charge allows it to bind and travel with the positively charged ions of sodium, potassium, calcium, and others.

Bound with sodium, the combination forms sodium chloride responsible for maintaining fluid balance and osmolality. When sodium and chloride are retained, so is water; when sodium and chloride are lost through the renal system, water is also lost. When the osmolarity is increased, more sodium and chloride ions are available compared to the percentage of water. When the osmolality is decreased, the number of sodium and chloride ions is also decreased compared to the percentage of water.

In the digestive system, chloride forms with the H$^+$ ion to make hydrochloric acid, aiding in digestion. It also plays an important role in maintaining acid/base balance.

Regulation of Chloride

Most of the required daily intake of chloride (3 to 9 g) is obtained through a healthy diet. This most commonly occurs through the use of table salt. However, chloride is also found in fruits, vegetables, cheese, milk, eggs, fish, and as a hidden source in canned vegetables or processed meats (see p. 52).

Maintaining Chloride Balance

Chloride is transported passively and due to its affinity for sodium, follows the active transport of sodium. Therefore, chloride levels in the body are increased or decreased proportionally along with changes in the sodium level. Sodium is directly affected by aldosterone, which indirectly affects chloride's relationship with sodium. As aldosterone is secreted, the kidneys reabsorb sodium and chloride becomes passively reabsorbed as it attaches itself to the sodium ion.

Chloride is exchanged for HCO_3 as the body maintains its acid/base balance. HCO_3 is retained to increase alkalinity and chloride is excreted. When the body needs a more acidic balance, HCO_3 is excreted via the kidneys and chloride is retained (see Chapter 30).

21 Hyperchloremia

<table>
<tr>
<td rowspan="2">HYPERCHLOREMIA</td>
<td>

INCREASED INTAKE/EXCHANGE

EXCESS SALT INTAKE WITHOUT WATER

HYPERTONIC IV FLUID ADMINISTRATION

METABOLIC ACIDOSIS

</td>
</tr>
<tr>
<td>

DECREASED LOSSES

HYPERPARATHYROIDISM

HYPERALDOSTERONISM

RENAL FAILURE

</td>
</tr>
</table>

Causes of Hyperchloremia
- Metabolic acidosis
- Hyperparathyroidism
- Hyperaldosteronism
- Hypernatremia
- Medications (i.e., salicylate toxicity, ion exchange resins)

Causes

Chloride has an affinity for sodium and an inverse relationship with HCO_3. These relationships are reflected in a chloride imbalance. High levels of chloride are related to excess sodium or decreased HCO_3 levels in the body. A level exceeding 106 mEq/L in the ECF constitutes a hyperchloremic condition.

Hyperchloremia can result from an increased intake orally or via administration of hypertonic IV fluids of sodium chloride coupled with a loss of water. Because of chloride's inverse relationship with HCO_3, hyperchloremia occurs in conditions of metabolic acidosis, when serum HCO_3 levels are low (see Chapter 30). Endocrine conditions, such as hyperparathyroidism and hyperaldosteronism, may be the cause of hyperchloremia, as well as hypernatremia, due to the ability of chloride to bind with sodium.

Certain drugs that contain chloride can be responsible for elevated chloride blood levels. Salicylate toxicity may cause hyperchloremia. Sodium polystyrene sulfonate, an ion exchange resin, is used in conditions of hyperkalemia and works by exchanging potassium for chloride in the bowel, eliminating potassium and retaining chloride (see above).

Manifestations

Hyperchloremia does not cause signs and symptoms related to a high chloride level. The chloride level is usually elevated when the sodium is high (i.e., hypernatremia) and the signs and symptoms would then relate to fluid overload (see p. 54). The heart rate may be tachycardic, blood pressure may be elevated, and dyspnea may be experienced, all secondary to the excess fluid.

Similarly, if hyperchloremia is due to an acidotic state, the signs and symptoms would be related to the acidotic state, not to the hyperchloremia. Signs and symptoms related to acidosis would be tachypnea, along with neurological manifestations of weakness, lethargy, and decreased cognition (see above).

Treatment

Treatment involves correcting the underlying condition. If hypernatremia is the cause, administering diuretics to assist in eliminating sodium will also help in removal of the chloride ion.

In states of acidosis, administering HCO_3 will help to correct the acidotic state and through competition for the connection with sodium, chloride will be eliminated. Lactated Ringer's solution may also be administered to help increase the HCO_3 level since the liver converts the lactate to HCO_3.

22 Hypochloremia

HYPOCHLOREMIA	DECREASED INTAKE
	Low salt dietary sources
	Exclusive D_5W IV fluid use
	Water intoxication (relative deficiency)
	INCREASED LOSS
	Diuresis
	Excessive vomiting (HCL loss)
	Metabolic alkalosis
	Fistulas
	Ileostomy
	NG suction
	Diarrhea

Causes of Hypochloremia
- Fistulas
- Ileostomy
- Nasogastric suction
- Vomiting
- Diarrhea
- Medications (i.e., loop, osmotic, or potassium–sparing diuretics)

Manifestations of Hypochloremia
- Agitation
- Irritability
- Hypertonicity
- Hyperactive reflexes
- Cramping/twitching
- Tetany

Hypochloremia + Metabolic Alkalosis = Decreased Respiratory Rate

Causes

Hypochloremia is defined as a serum chloride level of less than 98 mEq/L. It usually occurs in conjunction with low serum sodium levels or an elevated serum HCO_3 level.

Decreased Intake

A low serum chloride level occurs when intake decreases through a low salt diet. It may also occur with continuous administration of IV fluids without chloride such as dextrose in water. In rare situations, it may occur due to an extreme intake of free water.

Increased Loss/Decreased Absorption

An increase in chloride loss also contributes to hypochloremia. Chloride is lost through the renal and GI systems and through the skin with excessive sweating. Draining fistulas, ileostomies, or prolonged nasogastric suctioning without replacement of chloride can cause a hypochloremic state. Excessive vomiting and diarrhea are situations also related to chloride loss. When hydrochloric acid is lost from the stomach, a situation of metabolic alkalosis can occur as there is less competition for the HCO_3 ion with sodium. The loop, osmotic (mannitol), and thiazide (hydrochlorothiazide) diuretics may also bring about a loss of chloride through decreased absorption of water and electrolytes in the renal system (see p. 56). All losses contribute to decreased absorption.

Manifestations

Patients who suffer from hypochloremia manifest signs and symptoms associated with electrolyte imbalance, such as hyponatremia or hypokalemia. The nerves become excitable, causing a hypertonicity of the muscles and a hyperactivity of the deep tendon reflexes. The patient may experience cramping, twitching, and eventual tetany of the muscles. Agitation and irritability also accompany these situations (see p. 56).

If a state of metabolic alkalosis occurs, the body will attempt to compensate by retaining CO_2 via the respiratory system. This is manifested by a slow respiratory rate.

Treatment

As with many electrolyte and acid/base disturbances, treatment involves correction of the underlying cause. If a low salt diet is the problem, than salt intake should be increased. Broth or juices such as tomato juice are helpful.

If too much chloride is lost via the GI tract for various reasons, it may be replaced through IV fluids containing saline or oral supplements. Saline solution, not tap water, should be used for irrigation or flushing of any gastric tubes. If the hypochloremic condition is related to low potassium, potassium chloride may be added to the IV solution or administered orally if the patient is allowed oral intake.

23 Magnesium

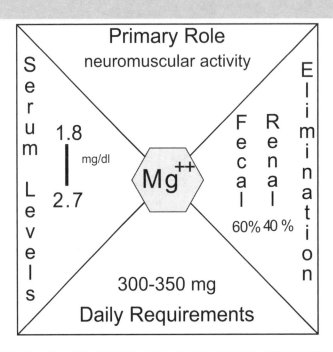

Primary Role
neuromuscular activity

Serum Levels

1.8 | 2.7 mg/dl

Mg^{++}

Fecal 60% Renal 40 %

Elimination

300-350 mg
Daily Requirements

Dietary Sources of Magnesium
- Seafood
- Meats
- Vegetables (e.g., dried beans, whole grains, peas, green leafy vegetables, broccoli)
- Chocolate
- Nuts, seeds
- Peanut butter
- Fruit
- Milk

Function

Following potassium, magnesium is the second most prevalent cation in the ICF. The normal concentration of magnesium is 1.8 to 2.7 mEq/L with very little found in the ECF and approximately 60% located in the bones. Magnesium is similar to calcium in that it is found either ionized in a physiologically active form (approximately two–thirds) or bound, primarily with albumin, and considered physiologically inactive (one–third).

Magnesium functions within the cell, activating enzymes for protein synthesis and carbohydrate metabolism. It helps to carry sodium and potassium across the cell membrane, helping to maintain electrolyte homeostasis. Magnesium has an effect on the parathyroid hormone, thereby influencing calcium levels. It also assists the body in the production of energy through the use and storage of ATP.

Magnesium acts as a transmitter of neuromuscular activity, particularly with the CNS, and helps with the contraction of heart muscle. Magnesium assists the release of acetylcholine at the neuromuscular junction, directly affecting muscles.

Regulation

A well–balanced diet supplies the necessary daily requirement (300 to 350 mg) for the body. Magnesium is found in various food sources such as seafood and meats; green leafy vegetables, which are rich in chlorophyll; dried beans; whole grains; peas; chocolate; and nuts (see p. 58). The body absorbs magnesium through the small intestine and excretes it via urine and feces.

Balance

A balance of magnesium is maintained in the body through absorption, excretion, or retention of the electrolyte via the GI tract or renal system. If magnesium levels are low, the body will absorb more through the small intestine. When levels are too high, more will be excreted by the kidneys through blockage of reabsorption in the proximal tubule and loop of Henle.

24 Hypermagnesemia

<table>
<tr><td rowspan="2">H Y P E R M A G N E S E M I A</td><td>

INCREASED INTAKE

INCREASED INTAKE WITH ANTACIDS

MAGNESIUM CATHARTIC ABUSE

IM / IV USE

</td></tr>
<tr><td>

DECREASED LOSS

RENAL FAILURE

ADRENAL INSUFFICIENCY

LEUKEMIA

HYPERPARATHYROIDISM

</td></tr>
</table>

Causes of Hypermagnesemia
- Medications (i.e., antacids, cathartics, magnesium sulfate, lithium)
- Dehydration
- Hyperparathyroidism
- Adrenal insufficiency
- Leukemia

Manifestations of Hypermagnesemia
- Warm, flushed appearance
- Diaphoresis
- Nausea/vomiting
- Drowsiness/lethargy
- Weakness and flaccid muscles
- Heart block and other dysrhythmias
- Respiratory and cardiac arrest
- Loss of deep tendon reflexes
- Depressed respiratory system (i.e., slow respirations, shallow respirations)
- Hypotension
- Bradycardia
- Coma

Causes

A magnesium serum level that is greater than 2.7 mEq/L is considered hypermagnesemia. The increased level occurs in the extracellular compartment and results from an increased intake or decreased excretion of magnesium. Though hypermagnesemia rarely occurs, an elevated level may result from an excessive intake of magnesium through magnesium–containing antacids or cathartics. It also may happen through an excessive administration of IV magnesium sulfate, particularly in the treatment of toxemia during pregnancy. Hypermagnesemia may also occur with the use of lithium (see p. 60).

The renal system is responsible for eliminating magnesium; therefore, renal insufficiency or renal failure will lead to elevated levels. Severe dehydration secondary to diabetic ketoacidosis (DKA) may cause a hemoconcentration of magnesium. A situation in which magnesium may transiently elevate occurs during stages of hyperparathyroidism when magnesium shifts from the bone to the ECF. Adrenal insufficiency and leukemia are also known causes of hypermagnesemia.

Manifestations

In states of hypermagnesemia, the release of acetylcholine is decreased at the neuromuscular junction, depressing neuromuscular function. This causes CNS sedative effects such as decreased reflexes. The patient may appear drowsy and lethargic. Diaphoresis and flushing occur. Muscles become weaker and flaccid as the serum magnesium level increases. Especially affected are the muscles of the respiratory system, which become depressed, resulting in slow, shallow respirations and the potential for respiratory arrest. The excitability of the cardiac membrane also becomes depressed and conduction decreases, resulting in bradycardia and hypotension. The possibility of cardiac dysrhythmias and possible cardiac arrest develop if the condition goes unattended (see p. 60).

Treatment

Treatment, as with many electrolyte imbalances, lies with correcting the underlying cause. Switching to a different antacid or stopping the use of laxatives may be necessary. Sodium inhibits renal tubular absorption of magnesium; therefore, IV saline solutions are helpful. Increasing the fluid intake along with diuretics may also help to flush out the excess. If the patient has a renal condition, dialysis may be necessary. They should also be cautioned against using magnesium–containing antacids and laxatives.

25 Hypomagnesemia

H Y P O M A G N E S E M I A	**DECREASED INTAKE** Alcoholism Anorexia Bulimia/purging Hyperalimentation
	INCREASED LOSS Diuresis diabetic ketoacidosis, primary aldostero- nism, diuretics Medications aminoglycosides, cisplatin, amphotericin

Causes of Hypomagnesemia

Decreased Intake	*Decreased Absorption*	*Excessive Loss*
• Alcoholism	• Laxatives	• Diuresis
• Anorexia	• Chronic diarrhea	• Diuretics
• Hyperalimentation	• Fistula drainage	• Burns/wounds
• Nasogastric drainage	• Antibiotics	
	• Digitalis	
	• Insulin	

Causes

Hypomagnesemia is a condition that results in a magnesium blood level of <1.8 mEq/L, but many patients do not experience symptoms until the serum level reaches 1.0 mEq/L. It occurs more frequently than hypermagnesemia and results from decreased intake or absorption of magnesium or excessive loss. Other electrolyte imbalances, such as hypokalemia, hypocalcemia, or metabolic acidosis, may enhance the effects of low magnesium (see above).

Decreased Intake

Alcoholics frequently suffer from hypomagnesemia due to a decreased dietary intake and, therefore, decreased absorption. There is also an increased loss through a high urine output or emesis with excessive alcohol use. Anorexic patients suffer from multiple electrolyte imbalances including hypomagnesemia. Patients who require long–term IV therapy during extended hospitalizations or hyperalimentation that are

> **Manifestations of Hypomagnesemia**
>
> Hypomagnesemia + Hypokalemia + Hypocalcemia = Neuromuscular Problems and Cardiac Dysrhythmias
>
> *Neuromuscular*
> - Hyperirritable nerves and muscles
> - Altered level of consciousness
> - Emotional lability/depression
> - Tremors/twitching/spasticity
> - Hyperactive deep tendon reflexes
> - Chvostek's sign
> - Trousseau's sign
> - Nystagmus
> - Seizures
> - Compromised respiratory system
>
> *Cardiac*
> - Prolonged PR, QT intervals
> - Prolonged QRS complex
> - Depressed ST segment
> - Flattened T with U wave
> - Premature ventricular contractions
> - Supraventricular tachycardia
> - Ventricular tachycardia
> - Ventricular fibrillation
> - Digitalis toxicity
>   Anorexia
>   Nausea/vomiting
>   Dysrhythmias
>   Yellow–green vision

not supplemented with magnesium may suffer from hypomagnesemia.

Decreased Absorption

People who overuse laxatives or those who take part in the binging/purging syndrome of bulimia do not allow enough time for the absorption of magnesium through the small bowel. Patients who suffer from chronic diarrhea or fistula drainage lose magnesium through the fluids contained in the lower GI tract. Patients with nasogastric suction may have decreased absorption in the intestine due to loss of magnesium from the upper GI tract.

Excessive Loss

Magnesium is lost through the renal system and affects anyone suffering from an excessive diuresis, such as that which accompanies DKA, hyperparathyroidism, or primary aldosteronism. Excessive or prolonged use of diuretics, particularly the more aggressive diuretics such as the thiazide or loop diuretics, results in an increased loss of fluid and, therefore, an increased loss/exchange of electrolytes including magnesium. Patients suffering from serious burns or wounds also lose magnesium through the injured area. The use of certain antibiotics, such as cyclosporine, amphotericin B, and aminoglycoside, may contribute to the loss of magnesium through increased urinary excretion. Chemotherapy regimens or digitalis and insulin are other commonly used drugs that affect the magnesium level (see p. 62).

Manifestations

Hypomagnesemia frequently occurs along with low potassium and calcium levels. This combined effect can result in cardiac and neurologic manifestations. The loss of magnesium affects the neuromuscular, central nervous, cardiovascular, and GI systems. Symptoms may go unnoticed or cause a life–threatening condition (see above).

Neuromuscular Manifestations

As magnesium leaves the body, more magnesium flows out of the cell. Depleting the intracellular level of magnesium leaves the cell weak, contributing to weakened skeletal muscles and hyperirritable nerves and muscles. Compared to hypermagnesemia, in which the muscles become weak, the muscles become hyperactive in hypomagnesemia, developing tremors, twitching, spasticity, and hyperactive deep tendon reflexes. Chvostek's sign (i.e., tapping the facial nerve and observing for facial twitching) and Trousseau's sign (i.e., compressing the upper arm and observing for carpal spasm) are positive. Nystagmus and seizures may occur. The respiratory muscles may also be affected, compromising breathing.

Central Nervous System Manifestations

CNS irritability involves an altered level of consciousness leading to confusion, personality change, depression, delusions, or hallucinations. Patients exhibit anxiety and irritability.

Cardiac Manifestations

When the magnesium level drops, the activity of the enzyme that propels the potassium/sodium pump decreases, causing a decreased flow of potassium into the cell. The cardiac muscle becomes irritable and dysrhythmias develop. Specific segments of the ECG become prolonged, such as the PR interval, QRS complex, and QT interval, or depressed, such as the ST segment, allowing for the interference of irritable beats.

Dangerous dysrhythmias can range from premature ventricular contractions to ventricular tachycardia and fibrillation. The risk of digitalis toxicity must also not be overlooked. A decreased magnesium level increases the retention of digitalis. Combined with low potassium, the cardiac muscle could be in severe jeopardy.

Gastrointestinal Manifestations

Patients with hypomagnesemia suffer from difficulty swallowing (i.e., dysphagia). They tend to have bouts of nausea and vomiting and become anorexic. This leads to a poor dietary intake.

Treatment

If the patient is suffering from low potassium and magnesium, replacing the potassium will not relieve symptoms until the magnesium level is brought to normal first. This is an important concept to remember with patients taking digoxin and diuretics. If the situation is severe, the replacement of magnesium should be done intravenously. If the level is not too low, oral supplements (i.e., magnesium oxide) may be used. As with any electrolyte disturbance, discovering the underlying cause for the imbalance must be accomplished.

1. What are the two main systems for regulating water levels?

(A) Low blood volume and sodium excretion

(B) Osmoreceptors and the renal system

(C) ADH and cellular dehydration

(D) The thirst mechanism and ADH

2. Which condition is the result of too much fluid in the vascular compartment?

(A) Edema

(B) Hypervolemia

(C) Hypovolemia

(D) Hypernatremia

3. Which of the following would be a dangerous outcome of ICF overload?

(A) Cerebral cellular rupture

(B) Hypervolemia

(C) Cellular dehydration

(D) CHF

4. Loss of body water along with a loss of sodium contributes to _____.

(A) Hypernatremia

(B) ICF overload

(C) Fluid volume deficit

(D) An increase in electrolytes

5. Which of the following is the most important cation in the ECF?

(A) Potassium

(B) Calcium

(C) Chloride

(D) Sodium

6. Hyperglycemia may cause which of the following conditions?

(A) Hypercalcemia

(B) Hypo–osmolar hyponatremia

(C) Hyperosmolar hyponatremia

(D) Hypocalcemia

7. How is potassium primarily excreted from the body?

(A) Cellular exchange

(B) Feces

(C) Urine

(D) Breathing

8. A greater loss of water compared to salt or an acute gain of salt compared to water results in which of the following conditions?

(A) Hyperkalemia

(B) Hypernatremia

(C) Hyponatremia

(D) Hypokalemia

9. Which of the following is a way to move potassium back into the cell during critical states of hyperkalemia?

(A) Diuretics

(B) Insulin and glucose

(C) Potassium supplement

(D) Increased dietary intake of potassium

10. Where is calcium primarily stored?

(A) Cells and fluid compartments

(B) Cardiac and smooth muscle

(C) Protein and small organic ions

(D) Bones and teeth

11. High chloride levels occur in combination with excess _____ and decreased _____.

(A) Sodium and HCO_3

(B) Potassium and calcium

(C) HCO_3 and sodium

(D) Parathyroid hormone and sodium

12. Which of the following electrolytes is the second most prevalent cation in the ICF?

(A) Sodium

(B) Magnesium

(C) Calcium

(D) Chloride

13. Parathyroid hormone helps to activate calcium from bone and is therefore responsible for which of the following?

(A) Hypernatremia

(B) Hypokalemia

(C) Hypercalcemia

(D) Hypocalcemia

14. What are Trousseau's and Chvostek's signs reflective of?

(A) Hypercalcemia

(B) Hypocalcemia

(C) Carpal spasm

(D) Decreased muscle excitability

1. The correct answer is D.

Both thirst and ADH are sensitive to osmolality and ECF volume. The other choices play a role in water balance or are an outcome of too little fluid volume.

2. The correct answer is B.

Too much fluid in the vascular compartment is known as *hypervolemia*. Edema is associated with fluid overload in the interstitial space. Hypovolemia is too little fluid in the vascular compartment. Hypernatremia is too much sodium and a probable cause of hypervolemia.

3. The correct answer is A.

Cells can rupture from too much fluid. The cells in the brain are the most vulnerable to this. Hypervolemia is too much fluid in the vascular compartment. Cellular dehydration is the opposite of fluid overload. CHF results from a weakened left ventricle, possibly from too much fluid in the vascular compartment, not fluid in the cells.

4. The correct answer is C.

When sodium is lost from the body, water follows, causing a deficit in fluid volume. Hypernatremia is a condition of too much sodium, not a loss. ICF overload is the result of too much fluid in the cells. An increase in electrolytes is vague and unrelated to what the question is asking.

5. The correct answer is D.

Sodium is the most prevalent and important cation in the ECF (135 to 148 mEq/L). Potassium is the most important in the intracellular compartment. Calcium is predominately found in the bones and teeth. Chloride is an anion.

6. The correct answer is C.

Increased glucose causes a hyperosmolar state. Water shifts to the area of increased glucose outside the cell, diluting the extracellular compartment. This causes hyponatremia in a hyperosmolar state. Calcium does not play a role in this situation and answer B is not associated with hyperglycemia.

7. The correct answer is C.

Potassium is primarily lost from the body via the renal system. Cellular exchange takes place during states of acidosis. Potassium is lost through feces, but only states of profuse diarrhea will cause a decrease in potassium levels.

8. The correct answer is B.

Hyponatremia is an excess of water compared to sodium. Hypo– and hyperkalemia refer to potassium.

9. The correct answer is B.

The combination of insulin and glucose helps drive potassium back into the cell. Diuretics will eliminate potassium through the renal system but will not assist in moving the ion back into the intracellular compartment. Potassium supplements and an increased dietary intake are only going to increase the potassium level, which is already elevated.

10. The correct answer is D.

Ninety–nine percent of calcium is located in the bones and teeth. The other 1% is found in the extracellular compartment and less than one–third of that is bound to protein. Calcium functions in the contraction of cardiac and skeletal muscle.

11. The correct answer is A.

Chloride loves to bind with sodium and works inversely with HCO_3; therefore, when sodium levels are high, chloride levels will also be elevated and HCO_3 levels will be decreased. Potassium is exchanged for chloride in conditions of hyperkalemia with potassium elimination taking place while chloride is retained. Hyperparathyroidism caused by elevated PTH levels may contribute to hyperchloremia, but sodium will not be decreased as suggested with answer D.

12. The correct answer is B.

Magnesium is the second most prevalent cation in ICF. Sodium is the most prevalent cation in the ECF. Calcium is a cation with somewhat equal concentrations in both the ECF and ICF, and chloride is an anion prevalent in the ECF.

13. The correct answer is C.

The parathyroid hormone helps activate calcium from bone so when excess parathyroid hormone is produced, it can be responsible for hypercalcemia.

14. The correct answer is B.

Hypocalcemia generates neuromuscular irritability manifested by a positive Trousseau's or Chvostek's sign. Hypercalcemia causes a decrease in neuromuscular excitability. Carpal spasm, elicited by occluding the arterial blood flow to the hand for ~3 minutes, is the positive indicator for Trousseau's sign. A facial twitch when the facial nerve is tapped is indicative of a positive Chvostek's sign. As a reminder, these signs are also positive with patients experiencing hypomagnesemia.

PART III
Acid/Base

26 Acid/Base

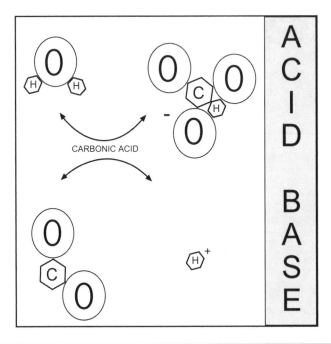

CARBONIC ACID

ACID BASE

---

pH Value and Acid/Base

$\downarrow$ pH = $\uparrow$ H$^+$ concentration = Acidosis

$\uparrow$ pH = $\downarrow$ H$^+$ concentration = Alkalosis

Understanding pH

The amount of acid or base in body fluid is reflected in the pH, the negative logarithm of the H$^+$ ion. The H$^+$ ion (acid) is needed for maintenance of cellular membranes and enzyme reactions, and minor alterations may affect metabolism and essential body functions. It travels in the body fluid as a volatile acid, H_2CO_3. It breaks down into H$^+$ and HCO_3^-. The volatile gas, CO_2, is expelled through breathing and the remaining part of the compound forms with other ions to make nonvolatile acids that are excreted in the urine. Nonvolatile acids such as the noncarbonic acids (hydrochloric,

phosphoric, etc.) are buffered and then eliminated via the renal system, not the respiratory system. Because acid/base balance is controlled primarily by the respiratory and renal systems, disorders affecting these systems will affect the pH balance. Many disease processes affecting the acid/base balance of the body may produce life–threatening alterations more damaging than the actual pathological condition.

The small concentration of the H$^+$ ion in the blood stream, 0.0000001 mg/L or 10^{-7}, is indicated as pH 7.0. An important concept to remember is that the greater the amount of H$^+$ ion, the more acidic the solution; the smaller the amount of H^+ ion, the more basic or alkaline the solution becomes. Because pH is based on a negative logarithm, the value lowers with higher H^+ ion concentrations and raises with lower H^+ ion concentrations; therefore, a low pH value equals an acidic solution and a high pH value indicates the solution is alkaline (see p. 70). The normal range for arterial blood is a pH level between 7.35 and 7.45. Death generally results if the levels fall below 6.9 or above 7.8.

Regulation of pH

The metabolic breakdown of proteins, carbohydrates, and fats produces H^+ ions that can combine to form acids. Three systems help to maintain acid/base homeostasis: buffers, the respiratory system, and the renal system. Buffers are chemicals that combine with an acid or base to weaken or neutralize it. Buffering is an immediate reaction to counteract the extreme changes in pH until other regulatory systems take over managing the situation (see Chapter 27).

The respiratory system expels CO_2 as a method for maintaining acid/base balance. Hypoventilation allows for the retention of H_2CO_3 and hyperventilation helps to expel the acid. Both are compensatory mechanisms that can act immediately to correct an acid/base imbalance (see Chapter 29).

The renal system is the slowest of the three systems to respond to an acid/base imbalance. Taking hours to days, it responds by excreting or reabsorbing the acid or base, whichever is required for regaining balance (see Chapter 28).

27 pH Regulation Through Buffering Systems

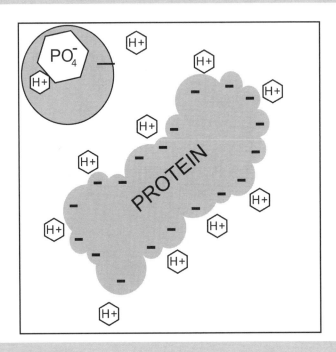

Buffering Systems

Proteins, H_2CO_3–HCO_3, phosphates, and the plasma potassium–hydrogen exchange control metabolic regulation of the body's pH. Some work outside the cell, some inside the cell, and others inside and outside the cell. The protein and HCO_3 buffering systems are immediately available and the most effective in maintaining the proper body pH.

Protein Buffers

Proteins are the most plentiful buffering system. They have a negative charge to buffer the H^+ ion and can release or bind with it. Therefore, they have the ability to function as an acid or base. Though proteins exist inside and outside the cell, most are primarily located inside the cell, making this an intracellular buffering mechanism. H^+ ions and CO_2 diffuse across the cell membrane to bind with proteins inside the cell, while albumin and plasma globulins act as the primary protein buffers in the vascular compartment.

Carbonic Acid–Bicarbonate

This buffering system is the largest in the ECF, particularly plasma and interstitial fluid. H_2CO_3 and HCO_3 are the major players working with the respiratory and renal systems. CO_2 and H_2O combine to form carbonic acid, $CO_2 + H_2O = H_2CO_3$, in the presence of the enzyme carbonic anhydrase, which catalyzes the reaction. As long as the rate of CO_2 being produced equals the rate in which it is expelled, the H^+ ion concentration will not change. If there is an excess of H^+ ions, the lungs can decrease the amount of H_2CO_3 through increased respirations, blowing off the CO_2 and leaving H_2O.

In the kidney, Na^+ is reabsorbed into the tubular cell and H^+ is secreted into the tubular fluid. In acidotic states, the renal system works by secreting excess H^+ ions to combine with HCO_3, resulting in CO_2 and H_2O. The water is eliminated via urine and the CO_2 travels to the tubular cell. With the help of the enzyme carbonic anhydrase, the CO_2 combines with H_2O in the tubular cell to make a new HCO_3^- ion and a free H^+ ion. The

HCO_3^- is then reabsorbed into the blood to combine with Na^+ and the lone H^+ ion starts another cycle in the tubular fluid.

If the situation is reversed (i.e., a state of alkalosis with a decreased number of H^+ ions), the H_2CO_3 will release H^+ ions to help decrease the pH to normal. The respiratory system will also attempt to slow respirations in an attempt to retain CO_2. To maintain a normal pH of 7.40, the HCO_3^--to-H_2CO_3 ratio must be kept at 20:1. The respiratory and renal systems work well together to keep this ratio. The respiratory system can work quickly to expel CO_2 and the renal system, though slower, easily reabsorbs or regenerates HCO_3.

Phosphate Buffers

The phosphate buffering system acts much like the H_2CO_3-HCO_3 system. Phosphates are highly concentrated in the ICF. Some of the phosphates act as weak acids to buffer stronger bases, and some act as a weak base to buffer a stronger acid. Buffering takes place predominately in the renal tubules where the greatest concentration of phosphates exist. The phosphate buffering system attempts to bring the pH back to normal by moving the H^+ from the plasma to the urine and eliminating the acid through urine.

Potassium–Hydrogen Exchange

These two positively charged ions move interchangeably in and out of the cell depending on excess. When there is an excess of H^+ ions in the ECF, they will move inside the cell for buffering and in exchange, the K^+ ion will move into the ECF. Therefore, it is important to note that changes in potassium levels can affect the acid/base balance in the body, as can a state of acidosis affect the potassium level.

Renal Regulation

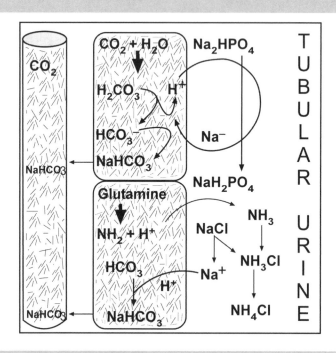

$$NH_3 + H^+ + NaCl + HCO_3^-$$
DISTAL

TUBULE

$$NaHCO_3 + NH_4Cl$$

The kidneys are effective in acid/base balance because they permanently remove the H$^+$ ion from the body. They also reabsorb acids or bases and produce HCO$_3$ ions. If the pH decreases, indicating a state of acidosis, the kidneys will conserve or make new HCO$_3$ and excrete an acidic urine. Conversely, if the pH rises, indicating a state of alkalosis, the kidneys will reabsorb the H$^+$ ion and excrete a more alkaline urine. Unlike the respiratory system, which can affect the pH in minutes, the renal processes are slow, taking hours to days to effectively regulate the pH; however, the effects of this system can last longer than other systems.

Hydrogen and Bicarbonate

In the proximal tubule, the H^+ ion is secreted into the fluid to combine with HCO_3. This combination, H_2CO_3, then forms CO_2 and H_2O. The H_2O is eliminated with the urine, and the CO_2 diffuses into the tubular cell. The CO_2, through a carbonic anhydrase–mediated reaction, helps to create a HCO_3 and a H^+ ion and the cycle continues.

Tubular System

The urine pH is maintained between 4.5 and 8.0. To keep too many free H^+ ions from making the urine overly acidic and, therefore, too caustic to the urinary tract, phosphate and ammonia buffering systems exist. The phosphate system tends to work best with high concentrations of hydrogen. This is because phosphate is poorly reabsorbed and remains concentrated in the tubule, allowing for more hydrogen to be gathered for buffering. Ammonia ions, NH_3, once secreted into the tubular fluid combine with the H^+ ion to make ammonium, NH_4^+. Ammonium ions are effective buffers because they are lipid soluble and cannot cross from the tubular fluid back into the blood. The ammonium then combines with a Cl^- ion, forming ammonium chloride (NH_4Cl) and is excreted in the urine (see p. 74). This system takes several days to generate sufficient amounts of ammonia to adequately buffer the acid.

Hydrogen/Potassium

Hydrogen is exchanged for potassium in the cell as potassium leaves the cell and enters the plasma during a state of acidosis. Consequently, the amount of H^+ ions decreases while the potassium level increases in the ECF. Alkalosis has the opposite effect by decreasing potassium levels.

Acid Exchange

In a state of acidosis with excess H_2CO_3, the kidneys will help maintain balance within the system by excreting other acids in an attempt to keep the pH from becoming exceedingly abnormal. If a lack of H_2CO_3 exists, then the kidneys work to retain other metabolic acids to maintain a balanced pH. This compensatory response takes several days to become completely efficient.

29 Respiratory Regulation

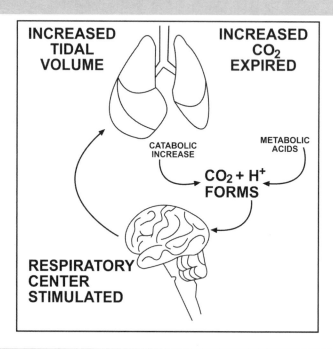

INCREASED TIDAL VOLUME

INCREASED CO₂ EXPIRED

CATABOLIC INCREASE

METABOLIC ACIDS

$CO_2 + H^+$ FORMS

RESPIRATORY CENTER STIMULATED

The respiratory system provides a quick response to an acid/base imbalance through control of the partial pressure of carbon dioxide ($PaCO_2$) in the arterial blood. When levels are elevated, CO_2 is a potent stimulus for ventilation. Carried by the RBC, CO_2 readily diffuses across the blood brain barrier, reacting with H_2O to form H_2CO_3 which in turn splits into HCO_3 and H^+.

It is the H^+ ion that is responsible for stimulating the respiratory drive. Increased amounts of H^+ cause an increase in respirations and a decreased amount of H^+ results in decreased respirations. As ventilation increases, CO_2 is blown off, leaving a decreased amount of CO_2 available to bond with H_2O. If acid is required for balancing the pH, a decreased respiratory rate will help retain CO_2.

The body compensates with the various forms of nonvolatile acid to maintain proper pH balance. In situations of inadequate oxygen delivery, lactic acid develops from the anaerobic metabolism of glucose. If a heavy load of lactic acid is circulating in the blood stream, the body will attempt to balance this increased acid-to-base ratio by eliminating CO_2 through an increased respiratory rate. The only way the respiratory system can remove acids is through the elimination of CO_2 from H_2CO_3. It cannot remove other acids. It is important to note that compensating for the increased acid does not correct the problem. If another acid is prevalent in the body, the respiratory system will eliminate the CO_2 in an attempt to compensate for the low pH and keep the pH from becoming dangerously low. The level of the particular acid initially responsible for the low pH, however, remains unchanged until other buffering mechanisms can remove the offending acid.

The respiratory system responds immediately to shifts in pH balance with hypoventilation for retention of CO_2 or hyperventilation to deplete CO_2. Though the response is rapid, there is a lag time before HCO_3 can reach adequate levels. Generally, the respiratory response reaches its maximum response in 12 to 24 hours. Also, the body can maintain a changed respiratory rate for only a limited amount of time before fatiguing.

30 Metabolic Acidosis

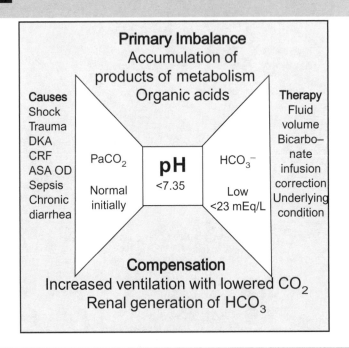

Primary Imbalance
Accumulation of
products of metabolism
Organic acids

Causes
Shock
Trauma
DKA
CRF
ASA OD
Sepsis
Chronic
diarrhea

$PaCO_2$

Normal
initially

pH
<7.35

HCO_3^-

Low
<23 mEq/L

Therapy
Fluid
volume
Bicarbo–
nate
infusion
correction
Underlying
condition

Compensation
Increased ventilation with lowered CO_2
Renal generation of HCO_3

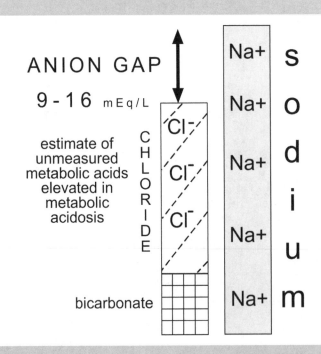

ANION GAP

9 - 16 mEq/L

estimate of
unmeasured
metabolic acids
elevated in
metabolic
acidosis

CHLORIDE

Cl^-

Cl^-

Cl^-

bicarbonate

Na+ s
Na+ o
Na+ d
Na+ i
Na+ u
Na+ m

Manifestations of Metabolic Acidosis	
Neurological	**Cardiac**
• Headache	• Decreased cardiac contractility
• Malaise	• Decreased cardiac output
• Weakness	• Dysrhythmias
• Fatigue	• Shock.
• Stupor/coma	
Sympathetic Nervous System	**Respiratory**
• Vasodilation	• Kussmaul's respirations
• Warm, flushed skin	
Gastrointestinal	
• Nausea/vomiting	
• Anorexia	
Hyperkalemia	

Causes

Metabolic acidosis results from a deficit in HCO_3 (<23 mEq/L) or an excess of noncarbonic acids. The pH is below 7.35 in metabolic acidosis.

Bicarbonate Deficit

A mechanism known to cause metabolic acidosis related to a HCO_3 deficit is a loss of HCO_3 through excessive intestinal secretions such as diarrhea, suction, or fistulas. A loss of HCO_3 can also occur through the renal system.

Excess Acid

Metabolic acidosis that results from increased acid levels can occur in situations involving an accumulation of lactic acid as in shock or cardiac arrest when anaerobic metabolism occurs due to insufficient oxygenation. Ketoacidosis can also result in metabolic acidosis, particularly with uncontrolled diabetes mellitus but also with excessive alcohol consumption, starvation, or ketogenic weight loss diets. Ingestion of methanol, ethylene glycol, or acetylsalicylic acid can produce extreme situations of metabolic acidosis and possible death. Decreased renal function also leads to a metabolic acidosis due to an inability of the kidneys to secrete H^+ ions into the urine or conserve HCO_3^-. This frequently occurs in the elderly as renal function decreases and the kidneys cannot eliminate an increased amount of acid that has accumulated or been ingested.

Hyperchloremic Acidosis

Hyperchloremic acidosis occurs with overtreatment of chloride–type medications, IV and hyperalimentation solutions, or increased absorption by the kidneys. Because HCO_3^- and Cl^- are both anions, the HCO_3^- concentration decreases when excess Cl^- ions are available. Ammonium chloride breaks down into NH_4^+ and Cl^-, allowing the ammonium ion to be converted to urea in the liver. This frees the Cl^- ion, allowing it to bind with available H^+ ions. The combination forms hydrochloric acid, resulting in a situation of HCO_3 deficit and increased acid.

Anion Gap

Evaluation of the anion gap is helpful in determining the condition responsible for the metabolic acidosis (see p. 78). It is used to identify the anions that are not measured. Conditions that result in a metabolic acidosis from excess acid create an increased anion gap. Normally, the sum of the cations is approximately equal to the sum of anions in the ECF. Sodium is the most plentiful cation in the ECF, and HCO_3^- and Cl^- are the most plentiful anions, with sodium usually outnumbering the HCO_3 and CL^- ions. Therefore, to determine the anion gap, the HCO_3 and Cl results are added together and subtracted from sodium, $Na^+ - (HCO_3^- + CL^-)$. A normal anion gap is 9 to 16 mEq/L.

Manifestations

A normal HCO_3 level is 23 to 27 mEq/L. When the pH falls below 7.35 and the HCO_3^- level drops below 23 mEq/L, a metabolic acidosis exists. Metabolic acidosis results secondary to an existing problem. Therefore, the characteristics of that particular disease process will be manifested along with the acidosis. Frequently, patients in metabolic acidosis will complain of fatigue, headache, weakness, or malaise. Anorexia, nausea, and vomiting may accompany the other symptoms. The SNS, responsible for vasoconstriction, loses its control over the skin vessels, allowing them to dilate and make the skin warm and flushed. Cellular membrane excitability becomes depressed, and as the condition worsens, the level of consciousness decreases to a stupor and eventual coma.

Cardiac contractility and output decrease and dysrhythmias develop as the pH continues to fall. Lactic acidosis begins to develop as ventricular function decreases and a shock state occurs. Acute metabolic acidosis is accompanied by respiratory compensation. The patient develops Kussmaul's respirations, a breathing pattern of deep rapid respirations in an attempt to eliminate acid via exhalation of CO_2.

Patients with chronic metabolic acidosis, such as that which accompanies renal failure, do not manifest all of the signs and symptoms as mentioned above due to the body's ability to compensate over time. In CRF, the problem of acidosis affects the skeletal system with the release of calcium and phosphate for buffering excess H^+ ions (see p. 79).

Treatment

Supplemental HCO_3^- may be helpful but not for conditions resulting in an increased ion gap. An example of this is a situation of lactic acidosis that occurs with cardiac arrest. This type of acidosis is often the result of inadequate oxygen perfusion. Adding more sodium HCO_3 to this scenario does not eliminate the oxygen problem and can cause hypernatremia and a state of hyperosmolality. It may also contribute to a decreased release of oxygen from the hemoglobin molecule, further complicating the lack of oxygen perfusion. The best treatment for metabolic acidosis is correcting the underlying problem and restoring fluid and electrolyte loss.

31 Metabolic Alkalosis

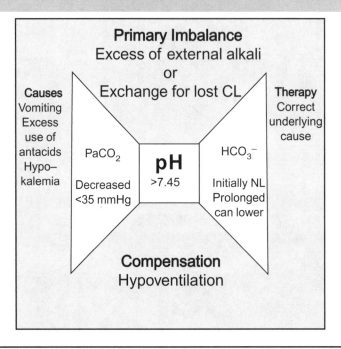

Primary Imbalance
Excess of external alkali
or
Exchange for lost CL

Causes
Vomiting
Excess use of antacids
Hypo–kalemia

Therapy
Correct underlying cause

PaCO$_2$
Decreased <35 mmHg

pH
>7.45

HCO$_3^-$
Initially NL
Prolonged can lower

Compensation
Hypoventilation

Manifestations of Metabolic Alkalosis

Neurological

- Mental confusion
- Neuromuscular irritability
- Hyperactive reflexes
- Tingling
- Tetany
- Seizures

Volume depletion

Hypokalemia

Respiratory failure

Cardiac dysrhythmias

Causes

Metabolic alkalosis can result from an excess of HCO_3^-, a deficit of acid, or perhaps a combination of both. The body's production and reabsorption of HCO_3 are usually maintained in a balance so that alkalosis does not occur. However, an intake of excess HCO_3 through antacids or overuse of HCO_3 products such as parental solutions containing lactate, hyperalimentation, or citrate with blood transfusions can increase the HCO_3 level above 27 mEq/L and the pH above 7.45.

Another possible cause is the removal of H^+ and Cl^- from the stomach through emesis or gastric suction, resulting in an excess of base. In situations in which K^+ is lost, such as through the use of diuretics or metabolic disorders, H^+ ion excretion is increased as the kidneys work to conserve K^+. The body also shifts the H^+ ion into the cell during conditions of hypokalemia and increases renal excretion of acid contributing to or causing metabolic alkalosis.

Manifestations

Patients with metabolic alkalosis resulting from a loss of body fluids through gastric suction, vomiting, binge–purge syndrome, or excessive diuretic use also manifest signs of volume depletion (postural hypotension) or hypokalemia. If the situation becomes severe, some may exhibit neuromuscular irritability. When the condition is acute, mental confusion occurs along with hyperactive reflexes, tingling, and tetany, leading to possible seizures. Respiratory failure, dysrhythmias, and eventual coma are manifestations of severe metabolic alkalosis with a pH greater than 7.55 (see p. 82).

Treatment

The compensatory mechanism for metabolic alkalosis is hypoventilation. By retaining CO_2, the body is increasing the acid content of the blood because CO_2 will combine with H_2O to make H_2CO_3. Treatment is again aimed at the underlying cause of the problem. If a chloride or potassium deficit exists, correcting the reason for the loss and supplementing with potassium chloride will help correct the problem. Patients suffering from an ECF loss will be given normal or one–half normal saline solution for replacement.

Respiratory Acidosis

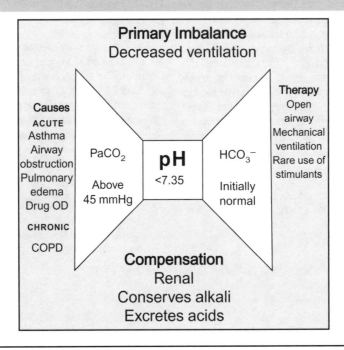

Primary Imbalance
Decreased ventilation

Causes
ACUTE
Asthma
Airway obstruction
Pulmonary edema
Drug OD

CHRONIC
COPD

$PaCO_2$
Above
45 mmHg

pH
<7.35

HCO_3^-
Initially
normal

Therapy
Open airway
Mechanical ventilation
Rare use of stimulants

Compensation
Renal
Conserves alkali
Excretes acids

Manifestations of Respiratory Acidosis

Neurological

- Headache
- Blurred vision
- Tremors
- Muscle twitching
- Vertigo
- Irritability
- Disorientation
- Lethargy

Cardiac

- Tachycardia
- Peripheral vasodilation

Respiratory

- Initial hyperventilation
- Eventual hypoventilation

Causes

Respiratory acidosis occurs when the pH value decreases below 7.35 and the PCO_2 level rises above 45 mmHg from hypoventilation. Alveolar ventilation becomes impaired, causing an increase in CO_2 and H_2CO_3. The H_2CO_3 dissociates, allowing for free H+ that contributes to the drop in pH. Acute and chronic conditions may be responsible.

Acute Respiratory Acidosis

Acute respiratory acidosis may occur with trauma that causes chest injury and impairs the respiratory system. A bronchial asthma attack, a sudden onset of pulmonary edema, drug overdose, airway obstruction, or head trauma causing a brainstem injury may also lead to difficulty breathing and the subsequent development of acidosis. The elderly have the potential to succumb to respiratory depression and, therefore, respiratory acidosis. As one ages, the ability to clear drugs efficiently through the renal system is decreased; therefore, taking medications, such as barbiturates, can cause a respiratory depression due to the decreased renal clearance.

Chronic Respiratory Acidosis

In long–term lung diseases such as emphysema or chronic obstructive pulmonary disease (COPD), areas of the respiratory system are permanently compromised in their ability to exchange CO_2 and O_2. Because such lung diseases are conditions that occur over time, the body adjusts to a permanently high CO_2 level (hypercapnia). The stimulus for respiration then stems from the state of hypoxemia and respiratory acidosis. In addition, the renal system continues to secrete H^+ and reabsorb HCO_3^- in an attempt at compensation. Patients with chronic respiratory disease can suffer from acute respiratory acidosis if O_2 is administered at a rate to suppress the stimulus for respirations. The patient's medullary respiratory center becomes used to the elevated PCO_2 levels. The respiratory drive then comes from the O_2 content in the blood. If the O_2 level is increased beyond the point of its normal stimulus, the patient's rate and depth of respiration becomes suppressed and the CO_2 content increases.

Manifestations

CO_2 readily diffuses across the blood brain barrier, causing neurological manifestations in the patient with respiratory acidosis. Headache occurs because the blood vessels in the brain dilate, which allows for more fluid to enter the vessel, increasing the cerebrospinal fluid pressure. Other neurological manifestations such as blurred vision, tremors and muscle twitching, vertigo, irritability, and disorientation occur secondary to the decreased pH of the cerebrospinal and interstitial fluid. Mild situations of acidosis result in flushed warm skin and weakness. In severe cases, lethargy progresses to coma if the pH remains unchanged. A decreased intracellular pH will affect the cardiac cells, causing tachycardia and other dysrhythmias. Peripheral vasodilation may occur, resulting in hypotension that may exacerbate the occurrence of dysrhythmias (see p. 84).

Treatment

Treatment is aimed at relieving the hypoxia and hypercapnia. If necessary, an airway must be established. Mechanical ventilation may be necessary for respiratory or neurologic failure. The kidneys cannot excrete H_2CO_3 but can excrete metabolic acids and will do so in an attempt to compensate the pH. They will also make and reabsorb HCO_3. The renal compensatory mechanism takes at least 24 hours to initiate and days to reach maximal effectiveness.

33 Respiratory Alkalosis

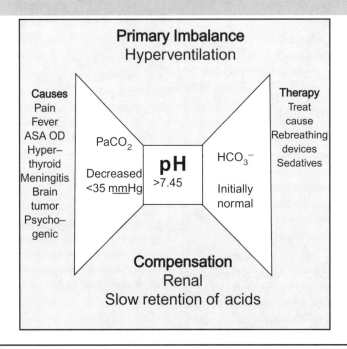

Primary Imbalance
Hyperventilation

Causes
Pain
Fever
ASA OD
Hyper–
thyroid
Meningitis
Brain
tumor
Psycho–
genic

$PaCO_2$
Decreased
<35 mmHg

pH
>7.45

HCO_3^-
Initially
normal

Therapy
Treat
cause
Rebreathing
devices
Sedatives

Compensation
Renal
Slow retention of acids

Manifestations of Respiratory Alkalosis

Neuromuscular Excitability

- Numbness/tingling
- Cramps/carpopedal spasms
- Decreased cerebral blood flow (i.e., lightheadedness, dizziness)

Sweating

Palpitation

Panic

Air Hunger

Causes

Respiratory alkalosis is the result of alveolar hyperventilation and a loss of CO_2 (i.e., hypocapnia) faster than the body can replace it. It is associated with a H_2CO_3 deficit, leading to a pH level greater than 7.45 and a CO_2 blood content of less than 35 mmHg. Respiratory alkalosis occurs secondary to hyperventilation when too much H_2CO_3 is expelled during expiration. The respirations are rapid and deep in hyperventilation. A common cause of respiratory alkalosis is panic attacks that result from high anxiety. A less common cause is gram–negative septicemia, which triggers the respiratory center in the brainstem to increase respirations to the point of hyperventilation.

Other causes are fever or oxygen deprivation such as that triggered in high altitudes. The early stages of salicylate toxicity also stimulate the medullary respiratory center of the brain stem to hyperventilate. An intentional cause for hyperventilation is through anesthesia or mechanical ventilation.

Manifestations

Symptoms of respiratory alkalosis are related to CNS irritability. Neuromuscular excitability is a manifestation of decreased calcium levels secondary to the binding of calcium to protein. This causes numbness and tingling (paresthesias) around the mouth, fingers, and toes. Positive Chvostek's and Trousseau's signs may be present. Cramps or carpopedal spasms may also be present. CO_2 easily crosses the blood brain barrier, causing vasoconstriction and a decreased cerebral blood flow. This results in lightheadedness and dizziness. Sweating, palpitations, panic, or air hunger may also be present (see p. 86).

Treatment

Treating the underlying cause and increasing the CO_2 level are of primary importance. Recognizing the initial problem is helpful since many conditions are short lived, such as panic attacks. Allowing one to rebreathe CO_2, such as blowing into a paper bag, is helpful for anxiety–induced alkalosis. The kidneys will attempt to retain H^+. However, this compensatory response takes several days.

34 Acid/Base Compensation

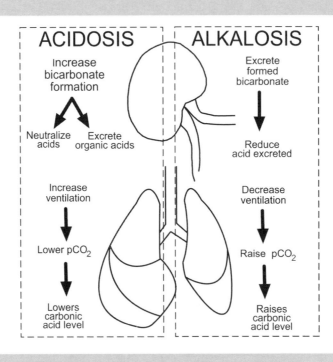

As mentioned previously, the body has built–in mechanisms to compensate for acid/base imbalances. Compensation, however, is not correction. It is the body's attempt to bring the imbalance back to normal. Unless the underlying condition is rectified, the imbalance will not be corrected. When compensating an acid/base disturbance, the system not responsible for the imbalance attempts to bring the blood pH back to normal.

Metabolic Acidosis

In metabolic acidosis, the respiratory system attempts to compensate by increasing the rate and depth of respirations through hyperventilation. When the pH drops below normal, the peripheral chemoreceptors stimulate the respiratory system in the brainstem. This increases the rate and depth of respirations in an attempt to blow off CO_2 and, therefore, lower the H_2CO_3 blood level. By lowering the H_2CO_3 level, there is less acid in the blood for the HCO_3 to buffer, helping to raise the HCO_3 levels. The arterial blood gases in a

patient with a compensated metabolic acidosis will show a slightly low or normal pH level of 7.35 to 7.40, a decreased HCO_3 (initial problem) level less than 23 mEq/L, and a decreased pCO_2 (compensatory response) of less than 35 mEq/L.

Metabolic Alkalosis

In metabolic alkalosis, the respiratory system again attempts to compensate. This time, it decreases its rate and depth of respirations through hypoventilation. Through decreased and shallow respirations, CO_2 is retained and the H_2CO_3 level is increased. Because the HCO_3 level is already increased, the increased level of H_2CO_3 helps bring the pH level back to normal. This is not an efficient mechanism for reversing metabolic alkalosis since the body needs oxygen and will not obtain enough through hypoventilation. Therefore, the respiratory system cannot respond in this manner for an extended period of time. The arterial blood gases of a patient with compensated metabolic alkalosis will show a slightly high or normal pH level of 7.40 to 7.45, an increased HCO_3 (initial problem) level greater than 27 mEq/L, and an increased pCO_2 (compensatory response) of greater than 45 mmHg.

Respiratory Acidosis

In respiratory acidosis, the kidneys work at excreting metabolic acid. The renal system is unable to eliminate H_2CO_3, but the ability to eliminate other acids helps to increase the HCO_3 concentration since less is needed for buffering the excess acid. This helps to move the ratio of HCO_3 to H_2CO_3 back to 20:1. The kidneys will increase the plasma HCO_3 level to great than 27 mEq/L. The arterial blood gases of a patient with a compensated respiratory acidosis will show a low or normal pH of 7.35 to 7.40, an elevated pCO_2 (the initial problem) greater than 45 mmHg, and a HCO_3 (compensatory mechanism) greater than 27 mEq/L.

Respiratory Alkalosis

In respiratory alkalosis, the lungs are excreting too much CO_2. The kidneys again attempt to compensate for the imbalance by decreasing the excretion of metabolic acid and, therefore, conserving acid. The renal system also attempts to decrease the HCO_3 concentration to less than 23 mEq/L. As more acid is circulating in the blood in lieu of the lost H_2CO_3, the HCO_3 concentration is used up with buffering. This tends to return the pH to normal. The renal system's compensatory response to respiratory alkalosis is infrequent since most of these situations are short lived. The arterial blood gases of a patient with a compensated respiratory alkalosis will show a slightly elevated or normal pH of 7.40 to 7.45, a pCO_2 less than 35 mmHg, and a HCO_3 (compensatory mechanism) less than 23 mEq/L.

35 Mixed Disturbances

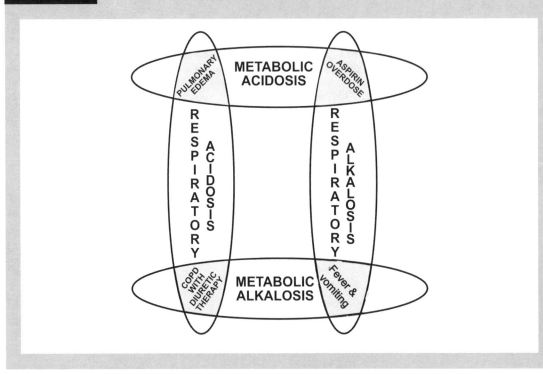

Acid/Base Imbalances

A primary acid/base imbalance occurs when there is an overwhelming amount of acid or base causing an imbalance with homeostasis. A metabolic acidosis occurs when the kidneys are not able to excrete enough metabolic acid or produce enough HCO_3 to equal the amount of acid. Metabolic alkalosis occurs when the kidneys produce too much HCO_3 and not enough acid is reabsorbed to counter the increased HCO_3.

In respiratory acidosis, too much H_2CO_3 is retained, causing a build up of CO_2 and not enough HCO_3 exists to compensate the increased H_2CO_3. Respiratory alkalosis occurs when too much H_2CO_3 is expelled as CO_2 and not enough metabolic acid is available to counteract for the lack of CO_2.

Mixed Disturbances

A mixed acid/base disturbance is an imbalance of both the respiratory and metabolic processes. This occurs when both the respiratory and renal systems demonstrate a primary imbalance with acid or base as a response to a disease process. How high or low the pH becomes depends on which system disturbance is most prevalent. There are numerous situations in which a mixed disturbance can develop. For example, COPD often manifests a respiratory acidosis. If the patient also suffers from diabetes mellitus and currently has a severe infection or has undergone the stress of surgery, a metabolic acidosis may also occur and then a mixed disturbance exists. Both the respiratory and metabolic systems are creating an acidotic situation.

Another example could be an elderly patient who is suffering from pneumonia, not exchanging air properly, and unable to expel secretions. The patient is given antibiotics and develops diarrhea from the medication. This patient could be in a respiratory acidosis from the pneumonia and metabolic acidosis from the diarrhea, a mixed disturbance. Frequently, a mixed disturbance occurs with patients suffering from cardiac arrest who develop a respiratory acidosis from hypoventilation and lactic acidosis from anaerobic metabolism.

Likewise, mixed disturbances can alter the alkaline status of the body. A patient connected to nasogastric suction loses acid along with the gastric secretions, causing metabolic alkalosis. If the patient is hyperventilating secondary to pain and losing CO_2, a respiratory alkalosis exists concurrently with the metabolic alkalosis.

Patients suffering from serious and chronic diseases suffer from mixed acid/base disorders. Mixed disturbances occur when both respiratory and metabolic disorders result in a condition of acidosis or alkalosis. Treatment depends on the situation and the condition.

36 Arterial Blood Gas Interpretation

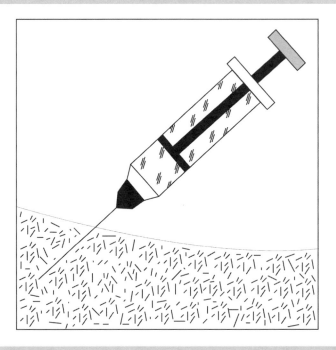

To interpret arterial blood gases for a patient, one must memorize the normal values, which are as follows:

pH   7.35 to 7.45
pCO_2 35 to 45 mmHg
HCO_3 23 to 27 mEq/L

The first step: Always look at the pH to determine acidosis or alkalosis.

pH   < 7.35 = acidosis
pH   >7.45 = alkalosis

The second step: Look at what is causing the imbalance. Is it the CO_2 or HCO_3^-?

pCO_2 <35 mmHg = alkalosis
pCO_2 >45 mmHg = acidosis
HCO_3 <23 mEq/L = acidosis
HCO_3 >27 mEq/L = alkalosis

The third step: Determine if compensation is occurring.

pH   7.35 to 7.40 = compensated acidosis
pH   7.40 to 7.45 = compensated alkalosis

Examples of Acid/Base Imbalances

Metabolic Acidosis (Uncompensated)
pH = 7.32
pCO_2 = 32 mmHg
HCO_3 = 14 mEq/L
Ex: Patient suffering from CRF.

Metabolic Acidosis (Compensated)
pH = 7.37
pCO_2 = 28 mmHg
HCO_3 = 18 mEq/L
Ex: pCO_2 has decreased through hyperventilation to decrease the amount of H_2CO_3 in the body.

Metabolic Alkalosis (Uncompensated)

pH = 7.52
pCO_2 = 48 mmHg
HCO_3 = 30 mEq/L
Ex: Patient losing acid through nasogastric suctioning.

Metabolic Alkalosis (Compensated)

pH = 7.44
pCO_2 = 48 mmHg
HCO_3 = 29 mEq/L
Ex: pCO_2 has increased through hypoventilation to increase the amount of H_2CO_3.

Respiratory Acidosis (Uncompensated)

pH = 7.33
pCO_2 = 55 mmHg
HCO_3 = 23 mEq/L
Ex: Patient with chronic obstructive lung disease.

Respiratory Acidosis (Compensated)

pH = 7.38
pCO_2 = 48 mmHg
HCO_3 = 29 mEq/L
Ex: HCO_3 has increased to compensate for elevated pCO_2.

Respiratory Alkalosis (Uncompensated)

pH = 7.50
pCO_2 = 30 mmHg
HCO_3 = 21 mEq/L
Ex: Patient with a hypermetabolic state, such as fever or sepsis.

Respiratory Alkalosis (Compensated)

pH = 7.44
pCO_2 = 32 mmHg
HCO_3 = 22 mEq/L
Ex: HCO_3 has decreased in an attempt to decrease HCO_3 levels compared to metabolic acids.

Respiratory and Metabolic Acidosis (Mixed Disturbance)

pH = 7.30
pCO_2 = 50 mmHg
HCO_3 = 19 mEq/L
Ex: Patient with CRF and COPD.

Respiratory and Metabolic Alkalosis (Mixed Disturbance)

pH = 7.50
pCO_2 = 32 mmHg
HCO_3 = 30 mEq/L
Ex: Patient hyperventilating from pain and connected to continuous nasogastric suction losing HCL acid along with gastric secretions.

1. The more H^+ ions in a solution, the more _____ the solution.

(A) Acidic

(B) Basic

(C) Salty

(D) Alkaline

2. Which following system is able to eliminate CO_2 to maintain acid/base balance?

(A) Renal system

(B) Protein buffering system

(C) Phosphate buffering system

(D) Respiratory system

3. In a state of acidosis, the _____ ion moves into the cell and the _____ ion moves out of the cell in an attempt to buffer the acidic state of the body.

(A) Potassium/hydrogen

(B) Sodium/chloride

(C) Chloride/sodium

(D) Hydrogen/potassium

4. If the pH rises, indicating an alkaline imbalance, how will the kidneys react?

(A) Eliminate the H^+ ion

(B) Attempt to hide the hydrogen ion inside the cell

(C) Reabsorb the hydrogen ion and excrete HCO_3

(D) Increase production of HCO_3

5. In a state of metabolic acidosis, the patient will manifest which of the following respiration patterns?

(A) Deep and rapid

(B) Slow and shallow

(C) Cluster

(D) Cheyne–Stokes

6. What is the compensatory mechanism for metabolic alkalosis?

(A) Hyperventilation

(B) Renal excretion of acid

(C) Hypoventilation

(D) Renal production and reabsorption of HCO_3

7. A patient with chronic lung disease becomes conditioned to an elevated _____ level in the blood.

(A) Oxygen

(B) Carbon dioxide

(C) Hydrogen

(D) Potassium

8. What condition occurs when too much CO_2 is expelled during expiration?

(A) Compensated respiratory acidosis

(B) Uncompensated metabolic acidosis

(C) Uncompensated metabolic alkalosis

(D) Compensated respiratory alkalosis

9. The following arterial blood gas (ABG) result of pH = 7.32, pCO_2 = 49 mmHg, HCO_3 mEq/L = 25 indicates which of the following conditions?

(A) Respiratory alkalosis

(B) Metabolic alkalosis

(C) Respiratory acidosis

(D) Metabolic acidosis

10. Which of the following ABG results indicate an uncompensated respiratory and metabolic alkalosis?

(A) pH = 7.50, pCO_2 = 32 mmHg, HCO_3 = 32 mEq/L

(B) pH = 7.30, pCO_2 = 50 mmHg, HCO_3 = 29 mEq/L

(C) pH = 7.45, pCO_2 = 45 mmHg, HCO_3 = 23 mEq/L

(D) pH =7.52, pCO_2 = 47 mmHg, HCO_3 = 29 mEq/L

PART III: ANSWERS

1. The correct answer is A.

Hydrogen is an acid; therefore, the more hydrogen ions in a solution, the more acidic the solution. The less hydrogen ions in a solution, the more alkaline the solution.

2. The correct answer is D.

Only the respiratory system can expel acid through respiration in an attempt to correct an acid imbalance. The renal system will produce HCO_3 as a buffering mechanism. The protein and phosphate systems will attempt to buffer excess acid in the body.

3. The correct answer is D.

The hydrogen ion (acid) will move into the cell in exchange for the potassium ion. This is an attempt to hide the acid inside the cell as the body attempts to buffer or eliminate the remaining acid.

4. The correct answer is C.

In an alkaline state, the kidneys will attempt to retain acid (hydrogen ion) and eliminate HCO_3. Eliminating the hydrogen ion or hiding it inside the cell will only increase the alkaline state. Increasing production of HCO_3 will also add base and increase the state of alkalinity.

5. The correct answer is A.

In a state of metabolic acidosis, the individual will attempt to rid the body of excess acid (carbon dioxide) through deep and rapid (Kussmaul's) respirations. Slow and shallow will only increase the amount of CO_2. Cluster breathing is an irregular pattern of cluster breaths with occasional periods of apnea. A Cheyne–Stokes pattern of breathing is a pattern of crescendo–decrescendo respirations accompanied by periods of apnea.

6. The correct answer is C.

The retention of CO_2 (acid) through hypoventilation will help increase the acid content of the blood. Hyperventilation will only increase the alkaline state by eliminating CO_2. Eliminating the H^+ ion (acid) through the renal system or retaining HCO_3 (base) will also only increase the alkalinity.

7. The correct answer is B.

Alveolar ventilation is impaired in the patient with chronic lung disease. This causes an increase in CO_2. The medullary system becomes accustomed to the elevated pCO_2 levels and the patient's respiratory drive can actually become suppressed from elevated O_2 administration.

8. The correct answer is D.

Respiratory alkalosis occurs when too much CO_2 is expelled, such as with conditions of hyperventilation. The renal system cannot expel CO_2 and respiratory acidosis is an accumulation of too much CO_2.

9. The correct answer is C.

The pH indicates an uncompensated state of acidosis; the CO_2 is elevated, indicating increased CO_2 in the blood; and the HCO_3 level is normal.

10. The correct answer is A.

Answer B is an uncompensated respiratory acidosis. Answer C is normal. Answer D is an uncompensated metabolic alkalosis.

PART IV
Organ Systems Control

37 Hypothalamus and Fluid Regulation

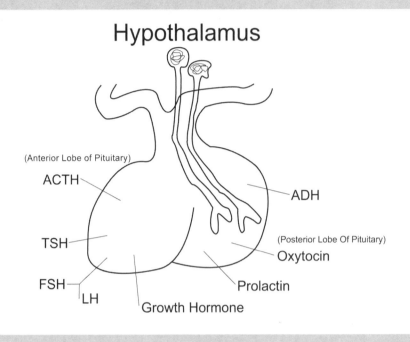

Hypothalamus

(Anterior Lobe of Pituitary)

ACTH

TSH

FSH

LH

Growth Hormone

ADH

(Posterior Lobe Of Pituitary)

Oxytocin

Prolactin

The hypothalamus is the most important organ responsible for maintaining homeostasis. Its control over respiratory, cardiovascular, stress, metabolic, and fluid and electrolyte balance is essential for supporting life. The hypothalamus is connected to and controls the pituitary gland, which has two lobes: the anterior lobe (adenohypophysis) and the posterior lobe (neurohypophysis). The anterior lobe is known as the *master gland* and conducts multiple functions through specialized cells that secrete specific hormones for particular metabolic roles. The posterior lobe, however, communicates with the hypothalamus in the regulation of fluid balance with the hormone ADH, or vasopressin. The hypothalamus synthesizes ADH, which is transported and stored in the neurohypophysis until its needed release for fluid regulation. A system of feedback loops is used to regulate the posterior pituitary gland to release ADH, which will affect the target organ producing the desired physiological response.

Thirst

Extremely sensitive osmoreceptors located near or in the thirst center of the hypothalamus are responsible for sensing the need for water. They have the capability to respond to changes in the osmolality of the extracellular compartment. When an increase in osmolality occurs, the cells dehydrate, which triggers the osmoreceptors to prompt the individual to take in water until the thirst center is satisfied. It is possible that the thirst center is connected to the storage and release area for ADH, accounting for the close relationship between the two.

Antidiuretic Hormone

The primary function of ADH is to regulate fluid volume based on the amount that can be absorbed via the renal tubules. ADH will help to replenish the fluid loss and regain homeostatic balance whether the initiator is decreased ECF or an increased sodium concentration.

38 Kidney Regulation of Electrolytes and Fluid

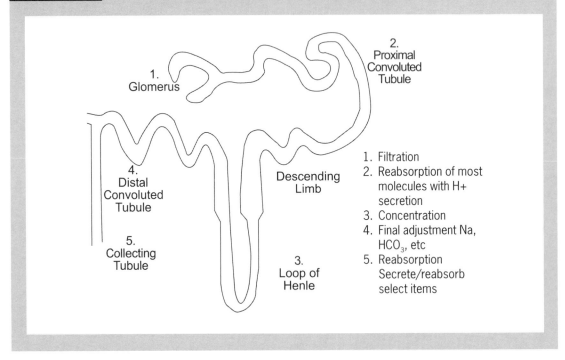

1. Glomerus
2. Proximal Convoluted Tubule
4. Distal Convoluted Tubule
Descending Limb
5. Collecting Tubule
3. Loop of Henle

1. Filtration
2. Reabsorption of most molecules with H+ secretion
3. Concentration
4. Final adjustment Na, HCO₃, etc
5. Reabsorption Secrete/reabsorb select items

The function of the kidneys is the removal and addition of substances to and from the blood through glomerular filtration, tubular reabsorption, and tubular secretion. Their ability to reabsorb and secrete electrolytes, maintain an acid/base balance, and conserve or eliminate water proves to be a remarkable system of checks and balances.

Glomerular Filtration

Glomerular filtration involves the filtering of fluids and solutes. Protein and blood cells are too large to pass through the glomerular filtration membrane barrier; therefore, the filtrate is a protein–free fluid with the same composition as plasma and in the healthy individual is iso–osmotic ~300 mOsm/L. Approximately 180 L of glomerulate filtrate is formed each day. Of this filtrate, 99% is reabsorbed and 1 to 2 L is considered urine output each day. Glomerular filtration is also helpful for the conservation of body fluids. Through constriction of the afferent arteriole, blood flow is decreased, which decreases the GFR, thereby conserving fluid.

Tubular Reabsorption

The kidneys have the ability to change the acid/base balance or composition of electrolytes in the plasma by changing the composition of the glomerular filtrate. Active and passive transport are the mechanisms of movement of molecules in the tubules. Some electrolytes passively ride on sodium (cotransport) as it is actively transported through the system. Other ions transport themselves through osmosis or diffusion in passive transport. As solutes become more concentrated on one side of the tubules and the other side becomes less concentrated, fluid will flow to the area of increased concentration. This helps to maintain a normal plasma osmolarity.

Concentration of Glomerular Filtrate As It Travels Through the Nephron

Urine formation starts as the filtrate formed in the glomerulus. It is protein–free plasma that will travel through the tubules and ducts of the nephron. Approximately 65% of reabsorption and secretion of electrolytes, vitamins, amino acids, etc. takes place in the proximal tubules of the kidney. Sodium and potassium are actively transported from the proximal collecting tubule into the capillaries. The movement of the two cations allows for negative ions such as Cl^- and HPO_4^{2-} to passively flow along to maintain electroneutrality. Hydrogen is actively exchanged for Na^+ in the proximal tubule then is allowed to combine with HCO_3^- to form H_2CO_3. H_2CO_3 readily breaks down into H_2O and CO_2, which diffuse and along with the enzyme carbonic anhydrase again form HCO_3^- and H^+. The HCO_3 combines with Na^+ and the H^+ is secreted to be again reabsorbed as H_2O.

The iso–osmotic glomerular filtrate passes from the proximal collecting tubule to the descending limb of the loop of Henle. As it moves down the loop, it meets with highly osmotic fluid in the medulla. The descending limb, under the influence of ADH, is readily permeable to water; therefore, the highly osmotic fluid initiates an osmotic movement of water out of the filtrate and the passive diffusion of Na^+ and Cl^- into the filtrate. The filtrate is hyperosmolar ~1200 mOsm/L as it begins to turn up the ascending limb of the loop of Henle. Unlike the descending limb, however, the ascending limb is impermeable to water. Solutes such as Na^+, Cl^-, and K^+ are readily reabsorbed here, but water cannot follow the ions. This makes the filtrate more dilute to the point of being hypo–osmolar. Traveling to the distal convoluted tubule, water continues to meet the barrier of impermeable tubules. Sodium and chloride reabsorption continues, contributing to the decreased osmolarity of the already dilute filtrate (see p. 100)..

As the filtrate travels to the late distal and cortical collecting tubules, aldosterone, a hormone secreted by the adrenal gland (see Chapter 8), exerts its affect on sodium reabsorption. This area is also a primary site for potassium excretion. Although potassium and sodium are excreted and reabsorbed along the journey through the glomerulus and nephron, the distal and cortical collecting tubules become the final place where the concentration of these two important electrolytes for the body is determined.

Fluid Regulation

During periods of dehydration or fluid excess, the kidneys work hard to maintain fluid balance. Whichever situation exists, the medullary collecting duct is where the fluid becomes highly concentrated or diluted. This also is where it becomes highly acidic or alkaline.

Fluid Conservation

ADH influences the regulation of fluid at the medullary collecting duct. If a need for fluid is sensed by the osmoreceptors, ADH is released by the neurohypophysis (posterior pituitary), sodium is reabsorbed, and the kidneys retain fluid.

Another influence on fluid balance is the renin–angiotensin–aldosterone system. When blood flow decreases, renin—an enzyme stored in the kidneys—is released. Through an enzyme–converting mechanism, it acts on angiotensinogen to become angiotensin I. Angiotensin I circulates to the lungs, meets with an ACE to become angiotensin II. Angiotensin II has the property of stimulating aldosterone to increase sodium reabsorption. In addition, it has the ability to vasoconstrict the efferent arteriole, allowing for an increased glomerular filtration pressure and maintenance of fluid volume.

Fluid Elimination

ANP is another hormone that has an effect over salt and water balance. Synthesized in the atrium of the heart, it is released when the muscle cells of the heart become stretched from too much volume. ANP aids in decreasing the amount of blood return to the heart through vasodilation of the blood vessels, which, in turn, affects the efferent and afferent arterioles of the kidney. This helps to increase the GFR. In addition, ANP inhibits the release of aldosterone and ADH, which prevents the reabsorption of sodium and H_2O.

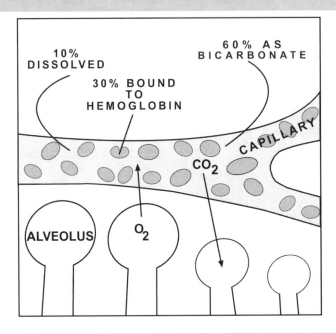

Carbon Dioxide

Through the process of breathing, a combination of oxygen and nitrogen gases enter the respiratory system. As the gases travel the vascular system, CO_2 travels the opposite pathway in exchange for oxygen. CO_2 diffuses into the capillary at the venous end and returns to the lungs via the pulmonary artery and arterioles. Once in the pulmonary bed, it diffuses across the alveolar–capillary interspace to enter the alveolus for expiration. Approximately 10% of CO_2 travels in its dissolved state in plasma. It is the dissolved CO_2 that is measured as the pCO_2 with a range of 35 to 45 mmHg. This range closely resembles that of the partial pressure of gases in the alveoli. Any increase in the amount of CO_2 can easily tilt the pH balance to an acidic state. Just as easily, any decrease in CO_2 can result in an increase in alkalinity. Of the remaining CO_2, 30% is attached to hemoglobin and 60% is transported as HCO_3. The dissolved CO_2 is carried to the alveoli of the lungs while the remaining diffuses into tissue spaces and capillaries.

Chloride Shift

CO_2 prefers to combine with hemoglobin (Hb–) in the RBC or with H_2CO_3. As mentioned previously, the $H_2CO_3^-$ easily ionizes to HCO_3^- and H^+. The hydrogen ion is allowed to combine with Hb– to form hydrogen hemoglobin, HHb, a buffer for acid/base alterations. If large amounts of HCO_3 are drawn into the plasma and a negative charge is needed in the RBC for equalization, Cl^- will move into the cell. This movement, referred to as a *chloride shift*, allows for increased amount of HCO_3 to move into the plasma to act as a buffering mechanism while chloride maintains electrical neutrality within the cell.

Within the respiratory system, attempts to rectify acid/base imbalances occur rapidly. The HHb molecule splits to release the H^+ ion so it can bond with HCO_3 again and form H_2CO_3. This combination rapidly breaks into H_2O and CO_2, which can be expelled during expiration to help decrease acid or kept to increase the acid balance. Chemoreceptors, sensitive to CO_2 changes, are located in the medulla of the brain. They will respond to an increased metabolic state by causing an increased formation of CO_2. In addition, if metabolism decreases, CO_2 formation will decrease. In this manner, the respiratory rate increases or decreases depending on the underlying cause.

Respiratory Fluid Loss

During expiration, H_2O is expelled along with gases. Though not in large amounts, if hyperventilation exists for a significant period of time, this loss of fluid can contribute to an already compromised fluid balance. In addition, the mouth, nose, and airway passages also become dried, making defense against debris removal and antimicrobial agents difficult.

Another method of fluid loss via the respiratory system is leakage out of the pulmonary capillaries. This is normally prevented through osmotic pressures and capillary hydrostatic pressure. However, fluid overload may cause fluid to leak into the alveoli and tissue interstitium, causing decreased diffusion of gases essential for breathing. This process will be discussed further in Part V.

Skin as a Barrier to Fluid Loss

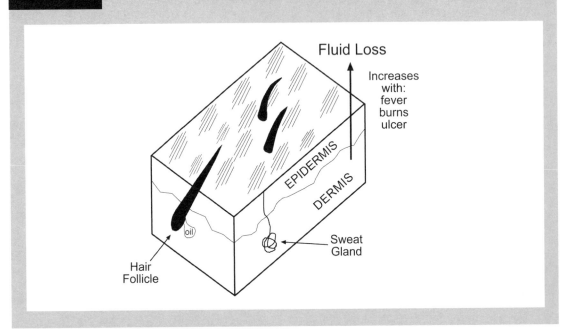

The skin is the largest organ in the body, protecting the musculoskeletal structure and internal organs. Known as the *integumentary system*, the skin—along with hair, nails, glands, and nerves—makes up an intricate structure that helps to regulate body temperature, fluid loss, production of vitamin D, and microbial defense. It comprises 20% of the body's weight. The skin has an elastic quality that allows for stretching. It is thick and tough in some areas, such as the palms of the hands and soles of the feet, while smooth and silky when forming the mucous membranes of the mouth and eyelids.

Fluid Loss Through the Skin

Along with its many other functions, the skin is waterproof, yet it allows for perspiration to help regulate body temperature. Through its peripheral thermoreceptors, the skin has an ability to trigger the hypothalamus for heat production and conservation when the temperature is low and evaporation when the temperature is hot. An increase in perspiration through the skin surface and mucous membrane linings aids in body water evaporation. Excessive perspiration, how-

ever, can affect the body's fluid balance and electrolyte status.

Burns are another source of rapid fluid loss through the skin. Fluid seeps out of open skin and also seeps into the tissues. The amount of protein loss affects the loss of fluid. Fluid shifts with the loss of protein, altered colloid osmotic pressure, and increased capillary permeability, causing edema.

Pressure ulcers and fistulas also affect water loss. Pressure sores form in vulnerable patients with compromised peripheral circulation or those unable to move and change positions normally. Compressing the skin so that the capillary pressure exceeds 25 mmHg occludes blood vessels in the tissue. Frequent repositioning helps to relieve this pressure, but ulcers begin to form when repositioning is not performed. Constant weeping from large pressure ulcers and fistulas can affect the body's fluid balance.

Trauma such as deep puncture wounds, facial lacerations, open compound fractures, and others cause an opening in the skin for blood loss. Major trauma can affect the body's fluid balance until replacement fluid has been administered and the skin repaired.

PART IV: QUESTIONS

1. Which of the following is a major hormone released by the hypothalamus/pituitary?

(A) Renin

(B) ADH

(C) ANP

(D) Creatine

2. The descending limb of the loop of Henle is readily _____ to water and the ascending limb of the loop of Henle is _____ to water.

(A) Permeable/impermeable

(B) Impermeable/permeable

3. Which of the following systems will expel CO_2 in response to metabolic acidotic state?

(A) Renal system

(B) Protein buffering system

(C) Phosphate buffering system

(D) Respiratory system

4. Which of the following is NOT a source of fluid loss through the skin?

(A) Deep puncture wounds

(B) Open compound fractures

(C) Exhalation

(D) Burns

PART IV: ANSWERS

1. The correct answer is B.

The hypothalamus/posterior pituitary releases ADH in response to an increased osmolality. Renin is initiated by the renal system in response to a need for vasoconstriction. ANP is synthesized in the atrium of the heart in response to an increased fluid volume. Creatine is a by–product of muscle catabolism.

2. The correct answer is A.

The descending limb is readily permeable to water, which helps with the passive diffusion of sodium and chloride into the filtrate. The ascending limb is impermeable to water, keeping the filtrate in a hypo–osmolar state.

3. The correct answer is D.

The respiratory system is the fastest responder to an acid/base imbalance through its ability to expel CO_2. The renal system is the slowest, taking days to weeks.

4. The correct answer is C.

Trauma such as deep puncture wounds, open compound fractures, and burns involve openings in the skin where fluid can escape. Fluid is lost through exhalation but is a function of the respiratory system and not the integumentary.

PART V
Fluid and Electrolyte Balance in Disease Processes and Nursing Implications

CAUSES	MANIFESTATIONS
PRERENAL	**STAGE 1**
HYPOVOLEMIA SHOCK ARTERIAL/ VENOUS OBSTRUCTION	90% OLIGURIC LOSE SODIUM GRADIENT BUN/CR RISE 1-7 DAYS
INTRARENAL	**STAGE 2**
GLOMERULONEPHRITIS NEPHROTOXIC AGENTS HEMOGLOBINURIA MYOGLOBINURIA IMMUNE/INFILTRATIVE	EARLY DIURESIS LARGE SHIFTS OF FLUIDS SEEN 1-3 WEEKS
POSTRENAL	**STAGE 3**
TUMOR OBSTRUCTION ENLARGED PROSTATE CALCULI TRAUMA	3-12 MONTHS 30% WITHOUT RECOVERY

Oliguria in Acute Renal Failure

Prerenal Causes	*Intrarenal Causes*
↑ Specific gravity	↓ Specific gravity
↑ Osmolality	↓ Osmolality
↓ Sodium content	↑ Sodium content
Little damage to kidney infrastructure	Damage to tubules
Autoregulatory mechanisms intact	Autoregulatory mechanisms NOT intact

Causes of Acute Renal Failure

Acute renal failure is related to a sudden decrease in the GFR causing a low urine output. It is treatable and reversible. The etiology of renal failure may be due to prerenal, intrarenal, or postrenal factors.

Prerenal Factors

Prerenal causes of acute renal failure occur as situations outside of the renal system that decrease pressure in the afferent arteriole and consequently restrict blood flow to the kidneys. Though compensatory measures help to maintain blood flow to the kidneys, an arterial pressure of less than 70 mmHg will cause most compensatory mechanisms to fail. Cardiovascular disorders; low blood volume; drugs causing vasoconstriction or peripheral dilation; or obstruction to the renal vasculature, such as clamping major arteries during surgery, are some of the factors related to decreasing the blood flow to the kidneys. If blood flow is restored in time, damage caused by these situations is minimal.

Intrarenal Factors

Intrarenal factors cause damage to the renal tissue and nephrons of the kidneys. The glomerulus may be the site of injury, such as with glomerulonephritis, but most commonly acute tubular necrosis (ATN) is the cause of acute renal failure. ATN can be caused by either prerenal or postrenal factors if they result in ischemia or nephrotoxic damage to the tubules. Nephrotoxic injury may be caused by aminoglycoside antibiotics or radiocontrast dyes. Hemoglobin released from damaged RBCs (caused by mismatched blood transfusions) or myoglobin released from crushed muscle cells (rhabdomyolysis) combined in a series of events have a direct toxic effect, causing damage to the tubular cell.

Postrenal Factors

Postrenal factors include the structures located distal to the kidneys. An obstruction to urine flow–whether located in the bladder, ureters, or urethra–can result in a backflow of urine to the kidneys, causing an increase in interstitial pressure and ultimately in the nephron. Prostatic hyperplasia, calculi, tumors, and trauma are some of the problems that can cause an obstruction to these urologic structures.

Clinical Manifestations of Acute Renal Failure

There are several stages in acute renal failure. The first stage is oliguria, which occurs in 1 to 7 days, depending on the initial insult. The second stage is diuresis and the third is the recovery stage.

Stage One: Oliguria

Oliguria Secondary to Prerenal Causes

Oliguria is the first stage of acute renal failure. Prerenal failure results from episodes related to decreased kidney perfusion (decreased pressure in the afferent arteriole) secondary to a decreased circulating blood volume to the kidney. Consequently, the body compensates through vasoconstriction and sodium and water retention. Therefore, oliguria secondary to prerenal causes in acute renal failure evidences urine with a high specific gravity, high osmolality, and low sodium content. There is little damage to the infrastructure of the kidney, and the autoregulatory mechanisms of the kidneys are able to compensate (see p. 110).

Oliguria Secondary to Intrarenal Causes

In contrast, the urine in oliguria related to intrarenal causes has a decreased specific gravity, decreased osmolality, the presence of casts, and increased sodium. These results are related to the damaged tubules that cannot respond to correction and, therefore, concentrate the urine.

Serum sodium cannot be conserved for long due to the damaged tubules and eventually levels fall. Care must be taken in evaluating the sodium levels, however, since they may actually be elevated but reflect a low value due to the increase in fluid (dilutional hypernatremia). Because retention of excess fluid volume is occurring at the same time, sodium should not be replaced. Volume excess may manifest as a bounding pulse, distended neck veins, or hypertension. If allowed to progress, CHF or pulmonary edema may develop.

Due to the damaged tubules, ammonia cannot be synthesized for H^+ excretion. Consequently, acidosis occurs due to accumulation of the H^+ ion. The respiratory system will attempt to compensate through rapid and deep (Kussmaul's) respirations in an effort to blow off CO_2. HCO_3 is available for buffering the H+, but supplies eventually diminish because the kidneys cannot replenish the quantity needed due to structural damage.

Several conditions exist to elevate the potassium level in acute renal failure. Potassium is normally lost through the urine. When output is impaired, potassium levels increase. In addition, if the acute failure is due to tissue injury, potassium is released from the damaged cells contributing to the elevated level. The exchange of intracellular potassium for H^+ in acidosis will also assist in elevating the potassium level (see Chapter 27).

The kidneys are responsible for activating vitamin D. Vitamin D is necessary for absorption of calcium from the GI tract. If the kidneys are not functioning properly, they cannot activate vitamin D, allowing for the development of hypocalcemia.

The BUN and creatinine levels also elevate, resulting in azotemia. These laboratory values are reflective of urea and nitrogenous wastes, which the kidneys normally excrete. Again, because the kidneys are not working to clear the wastes, the end products of metabolism accumulate.

Stage Two: Diuresis

Due to the increased urea concentration, an osmotic diuresis occurs and eventually the urine output increases. In addition, the nephrons have not regained normal functioning capacity and cannot concentrate the urine. These two factors combined contribute to a high urine output, which increases excessively to as much as 3 to 5 L/day. The loss of this amount of fluid may produce hypovolemia and dehydration. Electrolytes are now being lost through the high urine output, therefore, hypokalemia and hyponatremia may result. The patient may manifest signs of cardiac irritability and/or hypotension. The diuretic phase may last from 1 to 3 weeks before recovery begins to occur.

Stage Three: Recovery

As the diuresis stage ends, electrolyte, acid/base, and fluid balances begin to return to normal. It may take up to a year for the kidneys to regain complete function. Much depends on the overall health of the patient. If the patient is elderly and age has contributed to decreased renal perfusion and function, normal kidney function may never be regained.

Treatment/Nursing Implications

Monitoring the patient's fluid and electrolyte status during the oliguric and diuretic phases of acute renal failure is of primary importance. Accurate measurement of intake and output, along with daily weight, should be recorded. One should be alert for the signs and symptoms of hypervolemia and hypovolemia as the condition progresses through the various stages. Laboratory values and signs and symptoms of hyperna-tremia versus hyponatremia, hyperkalemia versus hypokalemia, hypocalcemia, and azotemia should be assessed. Acid/base balance must be monitored to avoid the progression of acidosis and the domino effect of electrolyte imbalance that follows. Prevention of infection through asepsis of invasive lines, tubes, and procedures is of paramount importance. Infection can be life threatening due to the compromised condition of the patient. Teaching the patient to comply with the treatment regimen, especially with an antibiotic regimen is important for complete recovery.

42 Chronic Renal Failure

```
         CAUSES        MANIFESTATIONS

        VASCULAR        FLUID BALANCE

  ARTERIAL BLOCKAGE      VARIABLE OUTPUT
  VENOUS OCCLUSION       HYPERVOLEMIA
  DIABETIC GLOMERULOSCLEROSIS   PERIPHERAL EDEMA
  post ATN

       INTRARENAL
                           METABOLIC

  GLOMERULONEPHRITIS
  TOXINS / MEDICATIONS     ACIDOSIS THAT IS ONLY
  IMMUNE                   SLOWLY COMPENSATED
      (GOODPASTURE'S)
  RENAL CELL CARCINOMA
  NEPHROSIS
                          ELECTROLYTES

       POSTRENAL
                          HYPERKALEMIA
                          HIGH PHOSPHATE
  TUMOR OBSTRUCTION       LOW CALCIUM
  CALCULI                 HIGH MAGNESIUM
                          DILUTIONAL LOW Na
```

Causes of Chronic Renal Failure

In CRF, also called end-stage renal disease, the glomeruli slowly sclerose, the tubules atrophy, and an interstitial fibrosis occurs. The nephrons eventually become damaged and can no longer function as they are replaced by scar tissue. Surprisingly, however, it takes up to 80% of nephron damage before altered renal function becomes clinically evident. The slow progress of this process may be caused by chronic obstruction from calculi, glomerulonephritis, or pyelonephritis. Long–term use of aminoglycoside antibiotics can result in nephrotoxicity. Diabetic nephropathy can cause CRF as well as hypertension and other vascular diseases.

Clinical Manifestations

End–stage renal failure is a multisystem disease. Multiple metabolic disturbances contribute to clinical manifestations with every system of the body (see p. 115). There is no cure for renal failure other than kid-ney transplant, provided the patient is a candidate for that procedure. Prior to that stage, dialysis helps to keep patients alive.

Fluid Imbalance

Unlike acute renal failure, which is classified by stages, CRF is progressive, beginning with a diminished renal reserve that progresses to renal insufficiency and ultimately results in end–stage renal disease. Even with a diminished renal reserve, the kidneys maintain a sufficient GFR to keep the serum creatinine and BUN levels normal. As the ability of the kidneys to concentrate urine diminishes, urine output increases and is one of the initial signs of the beginning of the disease process. Dehydration occurs if the condition goes unattended.

The progression of the disease eventually leads to a decreased number of functioning nephrons. Interestingly, the nephron is such a viable unit that dialysis is not required until almost 90% of the nephrons are lost. This is due to the ability of the remaining nephrons to

Metabolic Disturbances of Chronic Renal Failure	
Psychological	*Cardiovascular*

• Denial
• Anxiety
• Depression
• Psychosis
	• Hypertension
	• Congestive heart failure
	• Pericardial effusion
	• Myocardiopathy
	    Pericarditis
	    Atherosclerotic (heart disease, hyper–
	    lipidemia)

Neurologic	*Ocular*
• Fatigue • Headache • Sleep disturbances • Lethargy • Muscular irritability • Seizures • Confusion • Coma	• Hypertensive retinopathy
Pulmonary	*Gastrointestinal*
• Pulmonary edema • Dyspnea • Pneumonia • Uremic lung	• Anorexia • Nausea/vomiting • Gastritis/stomatitis • Peptic ulcer • GI bleed • Metallic taste in mouth • Nutritional deficiencies
Endocrine	*Reproductive*

• Hyperparathyroidism
• Thyroid dysfunction
	• Infertility
	• Sexual dysfunction
	    Azoospermia
	    Amenorrhea

Integumentary	*Metabolic*
• Pruritus/dry skin • Pallor/pigmentation changes • Ecchymosis/excoriations • Uremic frost	• Gout
Peripheral Neuropathy	*Hematologic*
• Paresthesias • Motor weakness • Restless leg syndrome	• Anemia • Bleeding • Infection

hypertrophy and compensate for the decrease in nephron numbers. As the disease progresses, the urine is no longer dilute; urine output decreases; and if intake exceeds output, hypervolemia occurs. The ability to clear urea and other metabolic products diminishes. The progression to end–stage renal failure is reflected as a creatinine clearance of 10 mL/minute compared to a normal of 85 to 135 mL/minute.

Metabolic Acidosis

The kidneys normally excrete a significant amount of acid on a daily basis. An impaired kidney, however, not only cannot excrete the H^+ ion, but it also cannot make extra HCO_3^- for buffering. The amount of HCO_3^- that exists is used up with the circulating acid. NH_4^+ excretion, another method for eliminating acid, is also decreased due to the lack of available ions (see

Chapter 28). Because CRF is a slowly progressing disease, the body has time to compensate for the imbalance more easily than with an acute acidotic situation.

Electrolyte Disturbances

Potassium

Oliguria is responsible for causing hyperkalemia. Potassium is primarily excreted from the body via the kidneys, and when little to no urine output exists, potassium is reabsorbed. In addition, due to the acidotic state, intracellular potassium is exchanged for the excess H^+ ion contributing more potassium to the elevated extracellular levels. The normal therapeutic range for potassium is 3.5 to 5.3 mEq/L. In renal failure, levels may rise as high as 7.0 or 8.0 mEq/L, contributing to life–threatening cardiac dysrhythmias and cardiac arrest.

Calcium and Phosphate

In an azotemic state, the GI system cannot absorb calcium due to the lack of activated vitamin D normally created by the kidneys. This results in hypocalcemia. At the same time, phosphate levels normally cleared by the kidneys rise because the kidneys are now functioning with a GFR below 25% of normal. Phosphate, inversely related to calcium, elevates as the calcium decreases. Due to the low calcium levels, the parathyroid hormone becomes activated and reabsorption of calcium from bone takes place (see Chapter 17). At the expense of the skeletal system, calcium levels are maintained. Eventually, however, hyperparathyroidism occurs due to constant stimulation of the gland. A precipitation of calcium–phosphate salts eventually accumulates in the soft tissues of the body, particularly around joints, causing arthritic pain. Consequently, the patient must consume a low phosphate and low protein diet.

Sodium

Initially, sodium is lost in CRF, causing an osmotic diuresis. This loss of water creates a dehydrated state. As oliguria occurs, sodium is retained along with water. This may contribute to a dilutional hyponatremia, or depending on the fluid balance, hypernatremic. A hypernatremic state may contribute to hypertension, edema, or CHF.

Magnesium

Magnesium, like other electrolytes, is excreted by the kidneys. The patient with CRF is at risk for increased serum magnesium levels. If the patient follows a low protein diet, decreased absorption of magnesium via the GI tract will help keep magnesium levels close to normal. In contrast, an increased intake of magnesium, such as overuse of antacids, can lead to a worsened state of hypermagnesemia. All products containing magnesium should be avoided by those with CRF.

Treatment/Nursing Implications

Neurologic

Neurologic changes occur as renal failure progresses and are often an indication that dialysis should be initiated. Though the cause is not completely known, it is believed that the toxic accumulation of waste products and electrolyte imbalances contributes to altered mentation. Assessment should include alertness, irritability, listlessness, or confusion. Observation for tetany, paresthesias, or muscle weakness should be conducted because these occurrences may be signs of electrolyte imbalance.

Cardiovascular

Hypotension may develop if fluid loss occurs; however, hypertension is more common secondary to hypernatremia and fluid retention. CHF may also result from the fluid overload or from left ventricular hypertrophy. If CHF occurs, basilar crackles and dyspnea may be present. Peripheral edema and distended neck veins may be present with fluid overload. A pericardial rub may be heard due to the pericarditis that develops from uremia. An irregular pulse may develop along with cardiac dysrhythmias from hyperkalemia. Monitoring vital signs and fluid and electrolyte balances are essential. Cardiac monitoring may be necessary if dysrhythmias develop. Antihypertensives, such as calcium channel blockers and ACE inhibitors, may be needed if sodium and fluid restriction are not effective. Blood pressure needs to be adjusted carefully because the kidneys have been dependent on a hypertensive blood flow driven through atherosclerotic vessels.

Patients become anemic due to the decreased production of erythropoietin, a hormone produced by the kidneys responsible for stimulating RBC production. Additional factors contributing to the patient's anemic state include a decreased RBC life span; hemolysis due to excessive intake of sodium in the RBC, causing the cell to swell and burst; bleeding from the GI tract; as well as frequent blood samples needed to monitor the client's condition. Hemoglobin and hematocrit levels should be monitored closely. Human erythropoietin may be available to treat the anemia.

Electrolyte

Potassium levels and the patient's cardiac status should be closely monitored. A potassium–restricted diet may be necessary. Diuretics or a cation–exchanging resin may help to eliminate excess potassium. If necessary, dialysis will help to adjust the potassium to a normal level.

Phosphate intake should be restricted and if levels are excessive, calcium–based phosphate binders may be given. Antacids containing calcium carbonate or aluminum hydroxide may be used to help bind phosphate and elevate calcium levels. Antacids containing magnesium will elevate the magnesium level and patients should be cautioned about over use of these products.

Checking for pitting edema, bounding pulse, and crackles at the lung bases are good measures for assessing fluid balance. A low sodium diet and fluid restriction are recommended for hypernatremia.

Respiratory

A predisposition to respiratory infections such as pneumonia or a uremic pleuritis develops. Pulmonary edema or dyspnea from fluid overload may occur and can be treated with diuretics or fluid removal with dialysis. Kussmaul's respirations will occur if the state of acidosis becomes severe. The patient should be assessed for shortness of breath and crackles, as well as deep rapid respirations associated with acidosis.

Gastrointestinal

Mucosal ulcerations, bleeding, and stomatitis secondary to the bacterial breakdown of urea are common. Anorexia frequently accompanies GI problems contributing to nutritional deficiencies. Diarrhea may result from hyperkalemia. Calcium absorption is impaired. Complications associated with the GI system are numerous and affect the patient's ability to eat and, thus, quality of life.

Protein restriction may help retard the degeneration of renal function. Adequate nutrition is important or the catabolism of proteins will occur. The breakdown of protein leads to increased urea, potassium, and phosphate levels; therefore, a low protein, high caloric diet is needed for the patient not undergoing dialysis. A higher intake of protein is allowed if the patient is undergoing dialysis.

Musculoskeletal

Renal osteodystrophy may develop in relation to the alterations in calcium and phosphate balance. The metabolic acidosis, decreased synthesis of vitamin D, and calcium and phosphorus imbalances combine to create this faulty bone condition that results in spontaneous fractures. Each of these conditions treated separately, such as lowering the phosphate level, supplementing calcium, administering an active form of vitamin D, and attempting to correct the acidosis, can help to decrease the destruction of bone.

Integumentary

Dry skin along with calcium and phosphorus deposits on the skin can lead to severe pruritus. Urea crystallizes on the skin when BUN levels elevate beyond normal, causing a condition known as *uremic frost*. Offering skin care with tepid water, using nondrying soaps, applying creams, and administering antihistamines provide relief for the itching.

Drug Therapy

Medications must be administered cautiously to patients with CRF. Almost all drugs are excreted partially or completely through the renal system. Because renal clearance is decreased, toxicity is a concern. Drugs may need to be administered in decreased dosages or less frequently to allow for renal clearance.

43 Disorders of Antidiuretic Hormone Regulation

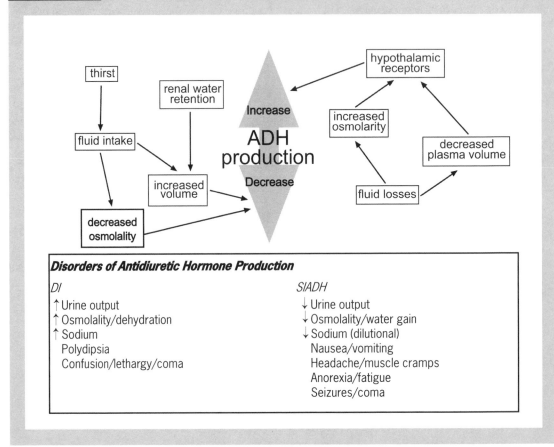

Disorders of Antidiuretic Hormone Production

DI
↑Urine output
↑Osmolality/dehydration
↑Sodium
Polydipsia
Confusion/lethargy/coma

SIADH
↓Urine output
↓Osmolality/water gain
↓Sodium (dilutional)
Nausea/vomiting
Headache/muscle cramps
Anorexia/fatigue
Seizures/coma

DI and SIADH are two conditions of abnormal ADH secretion that affect fluid and electrolyte balance. ADH is secreted by the hypothalamus to work on the renal tubules, increasing permeability for water and urea. When an insult to the cranium such as head trauma, tumors, or neurosurgery occurs, ADH secretion may be affected.

Diabetes Insipidus

Two types of DI can occur: neurogenic and nephrogenic. Neurogenic DI is related to the lack of release of ADH, even when hypertonic solutions that increase the plasma osmolality are administered. Nephrogenic DI occurs when the renal system cannot respond to ADH even when pharmacologic preparations of the hormone are administered.

Clinical Manifestations

Patients with DI lack the ability to concentrate urine; consequently, they produce vast quantities, sometimes as much as 15 L/day of dilute urine. Polydipsia generally accompanies the high urine output; therefore, if the patient is capable, enough water can be consumed to maintain an adequate fluid balance. Dehydration problems occur when the output is extreme and the person is unable to maintain the intake to equal the urine output or if the patient is unconscious and unaware of the need for fluid. An increased serum osmolality and hypertonic dehydration occur. Hypernatremia exists with DI due to the loss of water without the loss of sodium. Symptoms of thirst and confusion may occur. If the condition goes undiagnosed, the symptoms may progress to lethargy and seizures (see p. 118).

Treatment

Management of DI includes treatment of any underlying cause, replacement of fluid, and administration of ADH preparations. Such preparations must be given by nasal insufflations because they are destroyed in the GI tract if given orally.

Nursing Implications

Monitoring IV and PO fluid replacement is important. Measurement of intake and output along with daily weights is necessary. Serum electrolyte levels, especially sodium, must be closely monitored.

Syndrome of Inappropriate Antidiuretic Hormone

SIADH occurs when the feedback loop for the release and inhibition of ADH malfunctions. Even when serum osmolality is low and urine output should be increased, ADH continues to be secreted, resulting in clinical manifestations of water intoxication.

Clinical Manifestations

A dilutional hyponatremia is present along with a serum hypo–osmolality due to the abnormal reabsorption of water. Urine output decreases. Patients may complain of weight gain, headache, muscle cramps, anorexia, and fatigue related to the low sodium and excess water. If the condition persists with a sodium level of less than 125 mEq/L developing, nausea and vomiting may occur, leading to a greater electrolyte imbalance along with seizures and coma.

Treatment

Fluid restriction is the treatment for mild cases. Diuretics may also be necessary to eliminate excess fluid gain. If the sodium level is quite low, hypertonic saline solutions such as 3% NaCL may be required.

Nursing Implications

Assessing the level of consciousness is helpful, especially when looking for signs of hyponatremia. Accurate intake and output measurement, along with daily weights, are of extreme importance. Laboratory values should be monitored for electrolyte imbalance.

44 Respiratory Failure

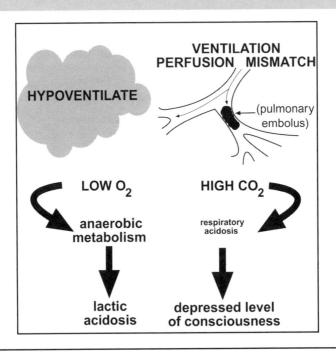

VENTILATION PERFUSION MISMATCH

HYPOVENTILATE

(pulmonary embolus)

LOW O$_2$ → anaerobic metabolism → lactic acidosis

HIGH CO$_2$ → respiratory acidosis → depressed level of consciousness

---

Respiratory Failure

Alveolar Hypoventilation = ↓PaO2 + ↑ CO2

V/Q Mismatch = Affected Ventilation + Unaffected Perfusion
OR
Affected Perfusion + Unaffected Ventilation

Shunt = Alveoli Filled With Fluid = No Gas Exchange

Causes

Respiratory failure occurs when the system is no longer able to exchange oxygen for CO$_2$. Either a situation exists in which sufficient oxygen is not available for transfer to the blood, resulting in hypoxemia, or CO$_2$ cannot be removed and is allowed to accumulate to dangerous levels, causing hypercapnia. It is not a disease in itself but the result of a disease—respiratory or otherwise. Two types of respiratory failure exist: hypoxemic failure and hypercapnic failure.

Hypoxemic Failure

Hypoxemia results from three different situations in the lung: alveolar hypoventilation, ventilation/perfusion (V/Q) mismatch, and intrapulmonary shunting (see above). As the term indicates, a lack or insufficient amount of oxygen exists in the blood for proper oxygenation. In hypoxemic failure, the PaO_2 level falls below 60 mmHg.

Alveolar Hypoventilation

Hypoventilation may be caused by a variety of conditions and results in decreased pO_2 and increased pCO_2 levels. Various conditions may cause hypoventilation, such as a decreased respiratory drive due to head injury or drug overdose; neuromuscular conditions affecting the respiratory muscles, such as amyotrophic lateral sclerosis or Guillain–Barré; chest wall dysfunction associated with trauma; or lung disease, such as COPD, cystic fibrosis, or acute respiratory distress syndrome. All affect the alveoli and gas exchange, causing hypoxemia.

Ventilation/Perfusion Mismatch

V/Q mismatch refers to discrepancies in ventilation/perfusion relationships. Although it is not an actual 1:1 ratio of ventilation to perfusion, overall, the ratio is close and varies slightly with certain areas of the lung. In situations of an accumulation of fluid in the alveoli, such as pneumonia, asthma resulting in bronchospasm, or the collapse of alveoli with atelectasis, air flow or ventilation is affected but perfusion to the alveoli continues unaffected. A pulmonary embolus is an example of the opposite. Due to the blockage of an embolus, blood flow would be interrupted, causing a perfusion problem but ventilation would continue unaffected. In such situations regardless of whether ventilation or perfusion is affected, there is a mismatch.

Intrapulmonary Shunt

Unoxygenated blood exiting from the heart is generally the result of a shunt. A shunt can result from an anatomical abnormality, such as a ventricular septal defect, where blood enters the right side of the heart and enters the left side without passing through the lungs. Another type of shunt is associated with pulmonary edema or acute respiratory distress syndrome. This type of shunt occurs when blood passes by the alveoli, which are filled with fluid, and cannot participate with gas exchange. Some respiratory conditions, such as pneumonia or adult respiratory distress syndrome, may result in a combination of a V/Q mismatch and shunting.

Hypercapnic Respiratory Failure

Hypercapnic respiratory failure is the inability to expel a sufficient amount of CO_2 (i.e., a failure in ventilation). Gas flow in and out of the lungs is normally adequate or exceeds the amount of ventilation needed to keep a normal $PaCO_2$ level. A person without lung disease not only has good ventilation at rest but is able to exercise, increasing the need for maximum ventilation without suffering from an increased $PaCO_2$ level and respiratory failure. When demand exceeds supply for a person with lung disease, that person will not be able to expel the CO_2 and respiratory failure ensues. Hyper-

capnic failure is evidenced by a $PaCO_2$ greater than 45 mmHg, which causes respiratory acidosis, and a pH level less than 7.35.

Clinical Manifestations of Acute Respiratory Failure

When a lack of O_2 or an increase in CO_2 occurs acutely, an emergency situation exists. Failure to meet the oxygen needs of the tissues can result in a major insult to the body. Early manifestations are related to the CNS. Confusion, irritability, anxiety, or combative behavior are warning signs of hypoxemia. If the oxygen deprivation continues, the body shifts to an anaerobic (without oxygen) metabolism, which consumes more energy than an aerobic (with oxygen) metabolism. In addition, the waste product of anaerobic metabolism is lactic acid, which requires HCO_3 for buffering. If enough HCO_3 does not exist, such as with patients suffering from CRF, then metabolic acidosis occurs along with respiratory acidosis, resulting in a mixed disturbance (see Chapter 35). When the body is in a state of acidosis, the compensatory mechanism of exchanging the H^+ ion for K^+ is initiated, contributing to a state of hyperkalemia (see Chapter 27).

Heart rate, respiratory rate, and cardiac output increase in an attempt to compensate for hypoxemia or blow off CO_2. Accessory respiratory muscles are used, and the normal inspiratory/expiratory ratio of 1:2 is increased to 1:3 or 1:4 in an attempt to expel the CO_2. The workload to keep up this increase is difficult, especially if lactic acid, which develops in an anaerobic environment, is already present. Respiratory compromise occurs and failure ensues.

Respiratory alkalosis may occur from hyperventilation and an excess loss of CO_2. If this occurs, the exchange of H^+ for K^+ will reverse, with H^+ exiting the cell and K^+ entering the cell, causing potential hypokalemia in the ECF, depending on the severity of the alkalosis.

Nursing Implications

Supplemental oxygen therapy is helpful for patients with a V/Q mismatch because not all of the areas of the lung are affected and additional oxygen is needed to compensate for the mismatched areas. Patients suffering from alveolar hypoventilation or a shunt problem will not benefit as easily from supplemental oxygen due to the fluid–filled alveoli that are unable to participate in gas exchange. Mechanical ventilation may be required for this type of patient with the addition of positive end expiratory pressure to help inflate the alveoli. Proper suctioning and maintenance of ventilator settings will assist the patient's respiratory status. The type of oxygen management depends on the condition causing the hypoxemia or hypercapnia. Arterial blood gas and electrolyte levels should be monitored closely.

Assessing the patient neurologically for hypoxic manifestations is important for early intervention. As the condition worsens, the patient's level of consciousness may become depressed. Respiratory assessment should include auscultation for air exchange in all lung fields; observation of accessory muscle use; and rate, depth, and character of respirations. Hemodynamic monitoring to assess blood flow and oxygenation is essential as well as monitoring lab values and arterial blood gas values. Cardiac monitoring is important for evaluation of dysrhythmias related to electrolyte imbalance and respiratory depression. Administering bronchodilators and corticosteroids will be helpful in opening the airways and decreasing swelling. Fluid balance should also be maintained.

45 Noncardiogenic Pulmonary Edema

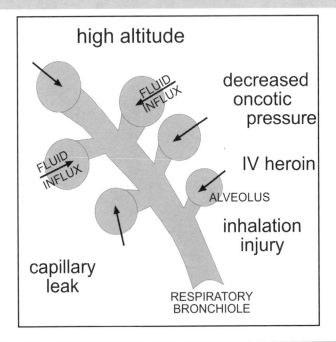

high altitude

FLUID INFLUX

decreased oncotic pressure

IV heroin

FLUID INFLUX

ALVEOLUS

inhalation injury

capillary leak

RESPIRATORY BRONCHIOLE

Noncardiogenic Pulmonary Edema Clinical Manifestations

- Feeling of impending doom
- Restlessness/agitation
- Dyspnea
- Tachypnea
- Dry cough leading to frothy, blood–tinged sputum
- Respiratory acidosis
- Bilateral crackles at bases

Causes of Noncardiogenic Pulmonary Edema

The source for pulmonary edema is frequently a failing cardiac system. Pulmonary edema, however, can result from numerous causes affecting the lung. Situations involving alveolar damage, such as septicemia, inhalation injuries with smoke or poisonous gases, or aspiration of toxic fluids, can cause increased capillary permeability in the lung bed.

Drug–induced injury from chemotherapeutic agents, heroin, inhalants, and others can also be the source of pulmonary edema. Other situations involving high altitude, head injury, lymphatic obstruction associated with malignant processes, or decreased colloidal osmotic pressure associated with liver or other wasting diseases can all be considered causes of noncardiogenic pulmonary edema.

Pathophysiology

The primary function of pulmonary circulation is to facilitate gas exchange. The pulmonary circulatory system has low resistance and low pressure. In comparison to the systemic circulation with an arterial mean pressure of 90 mmHg, the mean pressure of the pulmonary artery is 15 mmHg. This low pressure allows for greater increases in pulmonary blood flow during exercise and for the right ventricle's workload to be less than the left ventricle.

Fluid Balance

In the normal lung, a balance exists between the hydrostatic and oncotic pressures in the capillary beds. This balance prevents fluid from leaking from the capillary (see Chapter 7). If, however, the hydrostatic pressure increases or the colloidal oncotic pressure decreases, an interstitial pulmonary edema develops from the fluid leaving the capillaries and entering the interstitium. Initially, the lymphatic system will help transport excess fluid; however, as fluid continues to leave the pulmonary capillaries, excessive amounts begin to overwhelm the system, causing the fluid to push into the alveoli and resulting in pulmonary edema. This becomes detrimental to one's ability to breathe. Once fluid begins to enter the alveoli, gas exchange becomes impaired.

Gas Exchange

Oxygen and CO_2 are exchanged by diffusion (i.e., from an area of higher concentration to an area of lower concentration) in the pulmonary bed. The gases diffuse easily across the alveolar and capillary walls because these walls are only one cell thick. The exchange involves the movement of oxygen from the alveoli to the capillary and CO_2 from the capillary to the alveoli. The oxygen–rich blood is then circulated to the heart and eventually the tissues, while the CO_2 is removed from the alveoli during expiration. In pulmonary edema, the alveoli are filled with fluid and cannot contribute to the exchange of gases. CO_2 levels increase and oxygen levels decrease.

Clinical Manifestations

Dyspnea and tachypnea develop as the alveoli fill with fluid (see p. 124). The patient will complain of "lack of air" and a "feeling of impending doom." A cough develops with sputum that becomes frothy and blood tinged. Crackles are audible at the bases of the lungs. Arterial blood gas results will indicate respiratory acidosis, decreased PaO_2, and increased pCO_2 as the condition worsens.

Treatment/Nursing Implications

Oxygen administration is most important. Diuretics must be given to alleviate the excess fluids. Fluid and electrolyte balance must be maintained and any imbalances must be corrected. At times, mechanical ventilation with positive end expiratory pressure will be required to provide additional respiratory support. Identification of the underlying cause is necessary to determine the remaining treatment.

46 Heart Failure

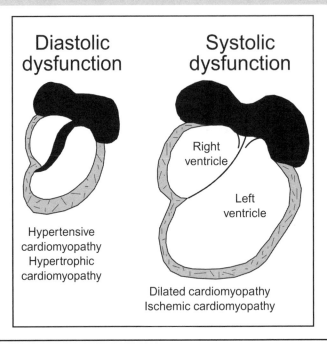

Diastolic dysfunction

Systolic dysfunction

Right ventricle

Left ventricle

Hypertensive cardiomyopathy
Hypertrophic cardiomyopathy

Dilated cardiomyopathy
Ischemic cardiomyopathy

Symptoms of Right-Sided and Left-Sided Heart Failure

Right Side

- Fatigue
- Jugular vein distension
- Peripheral edema (e.g., extremities, sacrum)
- Right upper quadrant pain (e.g., hepato–megaly, splenomegaly)
- GI bloating (ascites, nausea)

Left Side

- Fatigue
- Pulmonary congestion
- Pulmonary edema
- Dyspnea
- Orthopnea
- Paroxysmal nocturnal dyspnea

Causes of Heart Failure

Heart failure is an abnormal condition of the heart's ability to pump blood to meet the metabolic needs of the tissues. Heart failure results from multiple health problems or risk factors including obesity and elevated cholesterol levels that lead to coronary artery disease. Long–term diabetes mellitus causes severe damage to the vascular system and causes a predisposition to heart failure. Heart failure frequently occurs secondary to damaged cardiac muscle. Myocardial infarction, ventricular aneurysm, or myocarditis are problems that affect the contractility of the heart. Ventricular over-load, which is the result of increased blood return to the heart, may also result in CHF. Most commonly, heart failure results from hypertension associated with atherosclerosis of the heart and blood vessels from the sustained elevated high blood pressure levels. Whatever the cause, heart failure results in an increased workload for the ventricles. The increased workload of the heart eventually causes both the right and left ventricles to fail and improperly supply the body with oxygenated blood.

Numerous terms have been used to identify heart failure including *forward* and *backward*; *low* and *high output failure*; *systolic* and *diastolic*; *right sided* and *left sided*; or *CHF*, a more precise term when circulatory or pulmonary congestion is present. Systolic and diastolic and right sided and left sided are the current commonly used terms. Regardless of the description used to identify heart failure, the terms no longer seem different and tend to blend together as the disease progresses into a chronic condition. Emerging symptoms and system deterioration ultimately lead to a diminished quality of life and shortened life expectancy.

Pathology of Heart Failure

Systolic Failure

Systolic failure occurs when the left ventricle (systolic function) is affected by an event that affects the contractility of the cardiac muscle fibers, making the left ventricle unable to pump the blood effectively and empty completely. Attempts to pump blood from the left ventricle against the high pressured aorta fail, decreasing the left ventricular ejection fraction (i.e., the amount of blood ejected from the heart per beat, taking into consideration the entire amount of blood available per beat) and leaving blood in the ventricle, which increases the left ventricular end diastolic pressure. During subsequent cardiac cycles, the regular amount of blood is propelled from the right ventricle to the lungs to the left atrium and into the left ventricle. Already filled with blood from the previous cycle, the left ventricle cannot accept the quantity prepared for it. Eventually, blood accumulates in the pulmonary circulation, elevating the pulmonary capillary wedge pressure. Systolic failure is associated with dilated cardiomyopathy and ischemic cardiomyopathy along with other disorders.

Diastolic Failure

Diastolic failure occurs when the ventricles become unable to sufficiently relax and fill completely (diastolic function), resulting in a decreased amount of oxygenated blood returning from the lungs to the heart. Diastole is the heart's time to rest and passively fill with blood. Systole occurs when the heart contracts to pump blood to the tissues. In diastolic failure, the ventricles become stiff and noncompliant. Though the cardiac contraction may be effective, the high filling pressures and venous engorgement of the pulmonary and systemic vascular systems that the ventricles must pump against result in a noncompliant ventricle that does not fill properly. Diastolic failure occurs secondary to left ventricular hypertrophy, systemic hypertension, or aortic stenosis.

Left–Sided Failure

The terms *left–* and *right–sided failure* refer to the side of the heart with the initial impairment. Left–sided failure results when the heart can no longer pump a sufficient amount of blood to supply the tissues, causing blood to back up into the left atrium and pulmonary veins. Conditions that cause the left side of the heart to fail are many. Hypertension and myocardial infarction are two examples. Hypertension forces the ventricle to continuously pump against high pressures. This eventually leads to a hypertrophied muscle with poor contractility. Myocardial infarctions result in scar tissue that causes that particular area of the ventricular wall to lose elasticity and contractility. When the left side of the heart fails, blood backs up from the left ventricle to the left atrium and into the pulmonary bed, resulting in pulmonary congestion and edema. Dyspnea, orthopnea (i.e., shortness of breath in a recumbent position), paroxysmal nocturnal dyspnea (i.e., sudden, intermittent spasms of difficult breathing occurring at night), and a dry hacking cough (initially) are symptoms that accompany the pulmonary edema (see p. 126).

Right–Sided Failure

Because the right side of the heart works with the left, right–sided failure generally results from the left–sided problems; however, other conditions such as cor pulmonale (i.e., right ventricular enlargement secondary to lung disease), right ventricular infarction, or chronic pulmonary hypertension also contribute to right–sided failure. With blood backing up into the pulmonary bed, the right ventricle pumps harder to propel blood into the pulmonary artery. Eventually, the right ventricle fatigues, following the left ventricle. Blood backs up into the systemic venous circulation, causing jugular venous distension, peripheral edema, and vascular congestion of the GI tract, including the liver and spleen (see p. 126).

Clinical Manifestations

Dyspnea

Dyspnea is a common sign of heart failure. In the early stages, it occurs with activity. As the disease becomes progressively worse, dyspnea occurs more readily with less strenuous activities, eventually occurring at rest. Cardiac dyspnea is recognized in patients suffering from an engorged pulmonary vasculature and pulmonary interstitial edema, which affects lung compliance. When lung compliance is affected, the workload of the accessory muscles used to inflate the lungs increases. Breathing becomes more rapid and shallow, affecting the delivery of oxygen to these overworked muscles. Coupled with a decreased cardiac output, the shortness of breath contributes to fatigue, keeping the patient's activity at a minimum. Oxygen therapy becomes a fact of life along with restricted activity. Diuretics may be helpful with fluid overload.

Pulmonary Edema

Pulmonary edema occurs when the alveoli of the lungs fill with serosanguineous fluid. This situation can be a life–threatening manifestation of CHF. The patient may be agitated due to decreased oxygenation. Dyspnea, the use of accessory respiratory muscles, and an increased respiratory rate are common. Crackles and wheezes may be heard on auscultation and the patient may produce blood–tinged, frothy sputum. The patient may appear cyanotic and the skin becomes cool and clammy as vasoconstriction occurs in an attempt to keep the vital organs perfused. Tachycardia develops due to stimulation of the SNS sensing a decreased cardiac output. The blood pressure will either elevate or decrease depending on the severity of the edema and ability of the heart to maintain an increased rate. This condition requires immediate attention. Oxygen should be administered. Aggressive treatment with loop diuretics, such as furosemide administered intravenously, and fluid restriction is necessary. Morphine sulfate is helpful for decreasing the left ventricular end diastolic pressure as well as alleviating the patient's anxiety and feelings of impending doom. Inotropic drugs are helpful in increasing cardiac output and decreasing the increased SVR.

Peripheral Edema

Peripheral edema results from a local or generalized accumulation of fluid in the tissues. The lower extremities or sacrum of the sedentary or bedridden patient may be edematous, the liver may become engorged (hepatomegaly), the abdomen may retain fluid (ascites), or the spleen may retain fluid (splenomegaly). Diuretics are helpful for alleviating the excess fluid along with fluid restriction.

Electrolyte Imbalances

Hyponatremia may result from a dilutional affect or from overaggressive diuretic therapy. Hypomagnesemia may also occur with heavy diuretic use. Hypokalemia will result from excessive diuretic use, but hyperkalemia may occur from an acidotic state. Any electrolyte imbalance may lead to dysrhythmias in an already stressed and compromised heart.

Acid/Base Imbalance

Lactic acid, a product of anaerobic metabolism, is produced secondary to poor tissue perfusion. As lactic acid accumulates, metabolic acidosis occurs. In an attempt to compensate, the patient's respiratory rate will increase to blow off CO_2, potentially resulting in respiratory alkalosis. If the condition continues to the point of respiratory fatigue, CO_2 will accumulate, causing a mixed disturbance of metabolic and respiratory acidosis.

Treatment

Oxygen is a priority in the treatment of heart failure. If the patient is hospitalized, pulse oximetry monitoring to determine oxygen saturation is important along with the administration of oxygen. Diuretics, such as the loop diuretic furosemide, should be administered to help mobilize edematous fluid and reduce preload (ventricular filling pressure/the amount of stretch placed on the myocardial fibers). Potassium–sparing diuretics, such as spironolactone, may be used and are of help when used in combination with the loop diuretics. Vasodilators are also needed to reduce preload and afterload (i.e., the amount of peripheral resistance against which the left ventricle must pump), and inotropic agents are required to help strengthen the contractility of the heart. Morphine sulfate is frequently used to not only help decrease preload and afterload, but for the additional benefit of decreasing anxiety. The beta–blocking drugs are also helpful for blocking the SNS adverse effect of an increased heart rate. A low sodium diet (usually 2 g/day) is important to help minimize fluid retention.

Nursing Implications

Assessing signs of CHF should include looking for fatigue, activity intolerance, and restlessness due to decreased oxygenation. Monitor vital signs and oxygen saturation and assess for a rapid respiratory rate, dyspnea, and cough related to the accumulation of fluid in the lungs. Auscultate the lung fields for crackles. Evaluate arterial blood gases for acid/base balance. Note edema that may be present in the lower extremities. Cardiac monitoring is important for identification of dysrhythmias that may develop secondary to an imbalance of sodium and potassium electrolyte levels. Administer oxygen and medications as ordered.

⁴⁷ Diabetic Ketoacidosis

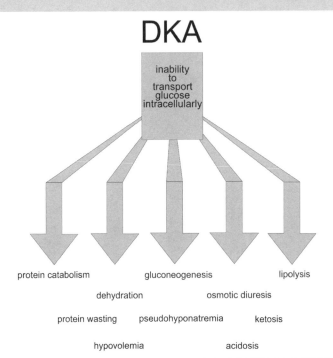

DKA

inability to transport glucose intracellularly

protein catabolism gluconeogenesis lipolysis

dehydration osmotic diuresis

protein wasting pseudohyponatremia ketosis

hypovolemia acidosis

Diabetic Ketoacidosis Clinical Manifestations
- Blood glucose levels >250 mg/dL
- Metabolic acidosis
- Fatigue
- Irritability
- Kussmaul's respirations
- Fruity "acetone" breath
- Flushed/dry skin
- Dry mucous membranes
- Increased thirst
- Urinary frequency
    Glucosuria/ketonuria
- Nausea/vomiting
    Acid/base imbalance
    Electrolyte loss
    Dehydration
      Hypotension
      Tachycardia

Diabetes mellitus is a group of heterogeneous disorders that affect carbohydrate metabolism and glucose homeostasis. There are two classifications of diabetes: type 1, which is characterized by pancreatic β–cell destruction and requires insulin replacement, and type 2, which is characterized by a secretory defect in insulin production and a resistance to the action of insulin on peripheral tissues. Type 2 diabetes can be controlled by diet and exercise. Under normal conditions, insulin is released into the blood stream continuously and increases with demands such as snacks and meals. Acute and chronic complications can happen with abnormal insulin release. Hyperglycemia and hypoglycemia are two extremes of blood glucose imbalance. DKA and hyperglycemic hyperosmolar nonketotic syndrome (HHNK) are two critical hyperglycemic states that will be discussed in this chapter and in Chapter 48.

Diabetic Ketoacidosis

DKA results from too little insulin in relation to an increased caloric intake or increased bodily stress. It primarily occurs with type I diabetes but can also take place with type II diabetes during times of severe illness or trauma, which cause an increased demand for insulin that cannot be met. When insufficient insulin is not available for glucose metabolism or carbohydrate metabolism, the liver metabolizes fats (lipolysis) to supply the body's energy needs. Keto acids are the product of this fat metabolism, and large quantities are released when carbohydrate stores are limited or cannot be accessed. An increased H^+ ion load develops as more ketones are produced than can be used, resulting in metabolic acidosis. With an altered pH, the body attempts to eliminate the ketones via urine, resulting in ketonuria. In an attempt to correct the state of acidosis, buffering cations, such as HCO_3 and potassium, are depleted with the excretion of keto acids and the acidotic state worsens.

The body continues to need energy and, as a compensatory mechanism, will generate glucose (gluconeogenesis) from the breakdown of protein. This results in a surplus of nitrogen and glucose that cannot be used due to the insufficient insulin levels. The plasma osmolality increases secondary to the increased state of hyperglycemia. This situation promotes the movement of ICF to the extracellular compartment, producing an osmotic diuresis. The increased loss of water contributes to a state of dehydration and electrolyte imbalances of potassium and sodium. In a state of acidosis, potassium is shifted from the intracellular compartment to the extracellular compartment in exchange for the H^+ ion, contributing to the lowering of potassium levels. A pseudohyponatremia may occur along with the ICF–ECF shift as water shifts to the extracellular compartment.

Clinical Manifestations

Clinical manifestations of DKA are related to the inability to utilize glucose for energy, resulting in fatigue and irritability (see p. 130). The blood glucose levels are greater than 250 mg/dL (normal fasting glucose levels are 80 to 90 mg/dL), and the state of acidosis is manifested by a low pH (<7.35) and a low HCO_3 level (<15 mEq/L). Kussmaul's respirations occur in an attempt to rid the body of excess acid by eliminating CO_2. One of the hallmark signs is a fruity or "acetone" breath, which results from the excess ketones in the body. The skin becomes flushed and dry along with dry mucous membranes due to the dehydration. In the early stages, patients will develop an increased thirst. If vomiting occurs, dehydration, acid/base balance, and electrolyte loss will be compounded. Hypotension and a weak rapid pulse also develop due to the low fluid volume and electrolyte imbalance. If left untreated, depression of the CNS will lead to shock and coma.

Treatment/Nursing Implications

Treatment of DKA involves correcting the fluid status, electrolyte imbalance, and acidosis. Fluid and electrolyte replacement is supplemented with IV solutions and based on plasma values. Most commonly, an IV solution of 0.45% or 0.9% NaCl is recommended to run at a rate of 1 L/hr until the blood pressure is stabilized and the urine output increases to 30 to 60 cc/hr. A bolus of short–acting insulin followed by continuous IV infusion of 0.1 U/kg/hr will help to stabilize the hyperglycemia and ketoacidosis. Care must be taken to gradually decrease the glucose levels. Once the blood glucose level approaches 250 mg/dL, dextrose is added to the IV solution to prevent the possibility of hypoglycemia. Potassium levels will elevate in the state of acidosis as potassium flows into the extracellular compartment in exchange for the H^+ ion, which moves into the cell. Therefore, the potassium levels may initially appear elevated; however, insulin drives potassium back into the cell and as the acidosis is corrected, potassium may need to be administered to correct any potential hypokalemic situations. Careful monitoring of the patient's neurological status, vital signs, cardiac status, lab values, and intake and output are essential.

48 Hyperglycemic Hyperosmolar Nonketotic Syndrome

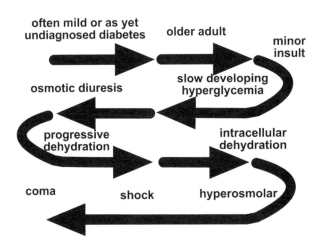

often mild or as yet undiagnosed diabetes → older adult → minor insult → slow developing hyperglycemia → osmotic diuresis → progressive dehydration → intracellular dehydration → coma ← shock ← hyperosmolar

---

Hyperglycemic Hyperosmolar Nonketotic Syndrome

- Blood glucose levels >600 mg/dL
- No acidosis
- Somnolence, weakness, lethargy
- Dehydration
    Dry mucous membranes
    Decreased skin turgor
    Orthostatic hypotension
- Left untreated
    Coma
    Death

Causes of Hyperglycemic Hyperosmolar Nonketotic Syndrome

A complication of diabetes that primarily affects patients with type 2 diabetes is HHNK. It is a medical emergency that affects individuals who can produce enough insulin to keep them from a state of acidosis but not enough to counteract the accumulation of excess glucose and the complicating high osmolarity and ECF loss. This event is frequently precipitated by a stressful event, such as infection, trauma, myocardial infarction, thrombolytic events, or acute pancreatitis. It has also been associated with certain medications, such as phenytoin and thiazide diuretics, and procedures, such as peritoneal dialysis. IV solutions containing a high glucose content, such as hyperalimentation, or enteral feedings have also been documented as precipitating HHNK. Older patients with a history of type 2 diabetes present with HHNK along with a recent history of polyuria and inadequate fluid intake.

Clinical Manifestations

This syndrome is manifested by a blood sugar usually greater than 600 mg/dL and plasma osmolality of 310 mOsm/L (see p. 132). The elevated glucose draws fluid from the cell to the extracellular compartment, resulting in dehydration that causes dry mucous membranes, decreased skin turgor, and orthostatic hypotension. In addition, the dehydration, if left untreated, affects the CNS, causing somnolence and eventual coma and death. HHNK and DKA are quite similar in presentation, but the main difference is the lack of ketoacidosis with HHNK.

Treatment/Nursing Implications

This condition is a medical emergency carrying a high mortality rate of ~50%. Treatment centers on restoring fluid balance from the high osmolar state to one of normalcy. Isotonic or hypotonic saline solutions are used for restoration; however, caution must be exercised to not administer fluids too aggressively because of the risk of causing cerebral edema due to a sudden rehydration of previously dehydrated brain cells. A guideline is to replace one–half of the estimated fluid deficit in the first 12 hours. Neurological assessment is an ongoing process, and measuring intake and output is extremely important. The patient's cardiac status should be monitored for dysrhythmias caused by the electrolyte imbalance. Electrolytes lost through the osmotic diuresis, especially sodium and potassium, must be replaced. Potassium also moves into the cell with the administration of insulin, compounding any state of hypokalemia that might exist. Frequent measurement of blood glucose results should be conducted, and short–acting insulin is administered as a bolus followed by continuous IV infusion of 0.1 U/kg/hr to decrease the high blood glucose. Once the blood glucose has dropped to approximately 250 mg/dL, dextrose is added to the IV solution to prevent hypoglycemia. Determining the underlying cause triggering the event needs to be determined along with educating the patient to prevent the event from happening in the future.

49 Burns

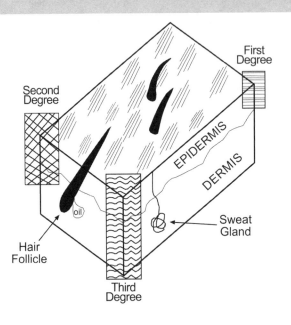

Burn Clinical Manifestations

Burn Injury

↓

↑Vascular Permeability = Edema + Protein Shift = ↓Colloidal Osmotic Pressure

+

Loss of Skin Barrier = Evaporation

↓

↓Circulating Volume = ↓Blood Pressure and ↓Cardiac Output

↓

↑SNS Stimulation = Vasoconstriction = ↑Heart Rate and ↑Cardiac Output

---

The physiologic changes accompanying burn injury are dependent on the degree and surface area of the burn. They range from first–degree minor injuries to fourth–degree predominately fatal injuries.

First-Degree Burns

First–degree burns destroy the outermost layer of the epidermis, but the skin remains intact. Blisters do not form, but erythema is present and the injured area is uncomfortable. First–degree burns occur from ultraviolet light exposure, such as sunburn or a brief exposure to hot liquid. Aspirin or acetaminophen helps to relieve the discomfort.

Second-Degree Burns

Second-degree burns involve a partial-thickness injury to the tissue and are classified as superficial or deep. The superficial second-degree burn takes 3 to 4 weeks for proper healing with the second-degree deep injury taking at least 30 or more days for complete healing to take place.

Superficial second-degree burns destroy the epidermis and lightly damage the dermis. The skin appears moist and weepy and blisters form. This type of injury may be caused by brief exposure to flame or hot liquids. Pain sensors remain intact; therefore, this type of burn is more painful than first-degree injuries. Generally, the site heals in 3 to 4 weeks provided infection does not occur.

Second-degree partial thickness burns destroy the epidermis, dermis, and epidermal appendages. Blisters form but do not have the normal fluid-filled appearance. Instead, they appear thin and paper-like. The injured area appears mottled, waxy-white, pink, or red in color. These burns result from flame or scalding liquids. With deep tissue destruction, pain sensors are destroyed; however, the area is surrounded by pain sensors in less damaged areas, which are extremely sensitive to the injury. In healthy people and without the complication of infection, this type of injury will heal in approximately 30 days. Skin grafting may be required.

Third-Degree Burns

Full thickness third-degree burns destroy the epidermis, dermis, and epidermal appendages. Damage extends the entire dermis, including the underlying subcutaneous tissue. The area of injury appears dry and leather-like because of the loss of skin elasticity. The color is a mottled brown or red. Edema is present and, combined with the leather-like skin, can constrict the tissue like a tourniquet. Unless an escharotomy is performed to relieve the pressure, the skin will burst or all circulation will be lost to the area. This type of injury occurs with prolonged contact with flame, scalding liquids, or steam. It may also result from electrical current or direct contact with chemicals. The pain receptors of the injured area are destroyed, but as with second-degree burns, there may be surrounding areas not as deeply burned that remain quite sensitive to pain. Skin grafting is required.

Fourth-Degree Burns

Fourth-degree burns are extremely serious injuries involving muscle and bone. The wound is dry; charred; and mottled brown, white, or red in color. There is no sensation to pain except for surrounding tissues that may have a lesser burned area such as second or third degree. These injuries occur from contact with an electrical current or prolonged contact with flame. Skin grafting is required and the limb may need to be amputated.

Clinical Manifestations

Serious burn injuries can initially result in hypovolemic shock, leading to hypoperfusion, acid/base and electrolyte imbalances, fluid loss, and organ failure. Initially, the increase in capillary endothelial permeability causes a massive shift of fluid from the vasculature. Sodium, water, and protein leak into the interstitial space, causing massive edema. As protein shifts from the vasculature to the interstitium, the colloidal osmotic pressure decreases, causing more fluid to shift. Second and third spacing take place as mediators of inflammation are released, causing vasodilation and compounding the hypotensive effect. As the circulating volume decreases, the blood pressure and cardiac output decrease. The compensatory SNS mechanisms take over, producing vasoconstriction via renin-angiotensin activation and ADH secretion (see Chapter 8). The heart rate accelerates to attempt an increase in the cardiac output. In addition to the fluid shifts, evaporation occurs through the lost skin barrier, also contributing to a loss of fluid, sometimes 200 to 400 mL/hr for someone critically burned. Complicating the sodium shift into the interstitial space, potassium also shifts to this area as it is released from the injured cells (see p. 134). Initially, hyperkalemia is present, as fluid resuscitation takes place; however, edema formation decreases and the capillary membrane is no longer permeable. This allows potassium to shift back into the cell. Sodium levels return to normal as fluid shifts back into the vascular space.

Nursing Implications

Assess for signs of decreased tissue perfusion and neurological manifestations of irritability or confusion, indicative of decreased cerebral perfusion. Monitor for cardiac dysrhythmias due to the electrolyte imbalances and fluid shifts that occur. Evaluate laboratory values for hyperkalemia and hyponatremia. The patient may manifest signs of an irregular heart rate, weakness, or diarrhea with hyperkalemia and twitching, seizures, nausea, and vomiting from hyponatremia. Monitor ABG results, assessing for metabolic acidosis. Strict intake and output along with daily weights should be implemented for evaluation of fluid loss. IV isotonic solutions should be closely monitored for proper fluid replacement. Wound care using strict aseptic techniques should follow the protocol of the burn unit.

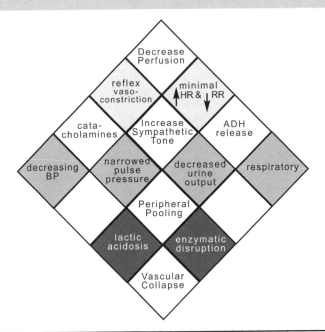

Decrease Perfusion

reflex vaso-constriction

minimal ↑ HR & ↓ RR

cata-cholamines

Increase Sympathetic Tone

ADH release

decreasing BP

narrowed pulse pressure

decreased urine output

respiratory

Peripheral Pooling

lactic acidosis

enzymatic disruption

Vascular Collapse

Clinical Manifestations of Shock

Stage I

- Alert and oriented x 3
- Restless/anxious/irritable
- Slight ↓ in blood pressure and ↑ in heart rate
- Narrowing pulse pressure
- Urine output normal or slightly ↓
- Acid/base normal

Stage II

- Vasoconstriction
- ↓ Cardiac output and blood pressure
- Anaerobic metabolism = lactic acid
- Acid/base = metabolic acidosis
- Hyperkalemia
- Possible cardiac dysrhythmias

Stage III

- Extreme hypotension
- ↑ Vasodilation = blood pooling in periphery
- ↑ Anaerobic metabolism = ↑ lactic acid production
- Compensatory mechanism nonfunctioning
- Multiple organ dysfunction
- Cardiac output unable to maintain tissue perfusion = cardiac and respiratory arrest

Shock is a syndrome of life–threatening hemodynamic imbalance leading to poor perfusion and an inadequate supply of oxygen and nutrients to the cells. Different classifications of shock exist, but the pathophysiology for all remains the same.

Stages of Shock

If detected early, shock can be reversed; however, as the shock state progresses, the chances of reversing the chain of events become impossible and death ensues. The first stage is compensation in which changes can be made to reverse the process. Stage II is the progressive stage, indicating that perfusion disturbance has increased and may lead to the third stage, the refractory stage or a condition that can no longer be reversed.

Stage I: Compensation

As stage I begins, the body's metabolic needs are still being met through adequate perfusion, but as the blood pressure decreases, compensatory mechanisms take over. Once the SNS is alerted to a decreasing blood pressure, peripheral vasoconstriction maintains blood flow to the major organs, particularly the brain and heart. A mild increase in heart rate helps to increase cardiac output, and dilation of the coronary arteries allows for an increased delivery of oxygen to the cardiac muscle.

Keeping the major organs perfused comes at a cost to other systems. Blood flow to the kidneys is decreased, which activates the release of renin which activates angiotensinogen to become angiotensin II, a potent vasoconstrictor. Aldosterone is stimulated to increase sodium reabsorption, and the release of ADH increases water reabsorption. The SNS hormones, epinephrine and norepinephrine, also cause vasoconstriction to the blood vessels. All help to increase blood volume to the heart and vital organs, but blood flow to other body systems is diminished.

Capillary hydrostatic pressure becomes decreased and falls below the colloidal osmotic pressure. This allows fluid to flow from the interstitial to the intravascular space, helping to increase blood volume and pressure.

Catecholamines are released to stimulate the liver to release its glycogen stores as the pancreas decreases its release of insulin. This allows an increased amount of glucose for the brain to use for energy during this time.

Clinical Manifestations of Stage I

During this stage, subtle changes occur that can be easily overlooked. The patient should be oriented to person, time, and place with clear speech but may appear somewhat restless and anxious (see p. 136). Irritability may be present. There may be a subtle drop in blood pressure, along with an increase in heart rate.

A characteristic sign is a narrowing of the pulse pressure (i.e., the difference between the systolic and diastolic pressures). The pulse pressure is an indicator of stroke volume, and a narrowed difference between the two pressures indicates a decrease in stroke volume. Urine output may remain normal or may show a slight decrease due to the activation of ADH. Acid/base balance should remain unaffected.

Stage I is the easiest stage to arrest the progression of the shock state. The difficulty with recognizing stage I is that most of the signs are subtle. Many may not be present, and the patient may easily slide into stage II before one is alerted to the possibility that problems exist.

Stage II: Progressive

The progressive stage occurs when the compensatory mechanisms fail to maintain an adequate cellular perfusion, and the initial signs of shock become more pronounced. Vasoconstriction becomes more apparent as the renin–angiotensin mechanism continues to respond to the low blood pressure. Cardiac output and blood pressure further decrease, resulting in tissue hypoxia, which causes anaerobic metabolism and the production of lactic acid. CO_2 cannot be removed due to poor blood flow; consequently, the level of acid in the body rises with the accumulation of intracellular H_2CO_3. The kidneys contribute to this worsening situation through impaired renal excretion of H^+. As the level of acidosis increases, electrolytes become imbalanced, particularly potassium, and affect myocardial contractility.

Clinical Manifestations of Stage II

Hypoxia dulls the SNS responses, so the patient is oriented to person but becomes easily confused. Speech may be slurred and the patient may complain of thirst, dry lips, and dry mouth. A decreased response to painful stimuli occurs. The skin begins to feel cool and appears pale as vasoconstriction becomes more intense. The systolic blood pressure continues to fall, and the pulse pressure continues to narrow. The heart rate becomes increasingly tachycardic and the pulse feels weak and thready. Due to all of the vasoconstrictive measures, urine output now becomes obviously decreased to approximately 20 to 30 cc/hr. The respiratory system attempts to decrease the acidosis by increasing respirations to blow off CO_2 and lower the H_2CO_3 level.

Stage III: Refractory

The third stage of shock is virtually irreversible. The compensatory mechanisms are no longer functioning, the blood pressure cannot be maintained, and a syndrome of multiple organ dysfunction (MODS) occurs. Every system is compromised and becomes dysfunctional. The cascade of effects is overwhelming, and the body is unable to recover.

Clinical Manifestations of Stage III

An anaerobic metabolism occurs secondary to a lack of oxygen, which contributes to the production of lactic acid and a metabolic/respiratory acidotic state. The SNS can no longer maintain its measures for vasoconstriction, and a loss of sympathetic tone allows blood to pool in the periphery. Blood also pools in the capillaries, creating a movement of fluid out of the vascular space, which furthers the hypotension. Cardiac output becomes too low to maintain cerebral, cardiac, respiratory, and renal perfusion. Underperfused and needing oxygen, the tissues suffer from the insult of a severe acidosis and cellular ischemia/death, leading to cardiac and respiratory arrest.

51 Types of Shock

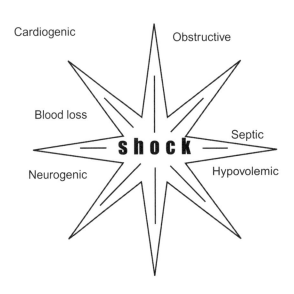

```
        Cardiogenic              Obstructive



        Blood loss
                          shock          Septic

        Neurogenic                  Hypovolemic
```

Categorizing Shock

- Cardiogenic shock = inability of heart to pump blood throughout the body
- Circulatory shock = loss of intravascular volume
      Hypovolemic
      Obstructive
- Distributive shock = loss of blood vessel tone
      Neurogenic
      Anaphylactic
      Septic

Shock Categories

Shock is generally classified into three categories (see above). Cardiogenic shock is the inability of the heart to pump blood throughout the body. Circulatory shock is the loss of intravascular volume and has two subclassifications: hypovolemic and obstructive. The third main classification is distributive shock, which includes subclassifications of neurogenic, anaphylactic, and septic shock. Regardless of the type of shock, the stages the patient goes through remain the same.

The compensatory mechanisms do not change because the end result for all types, if uncorrected, is a decreased perfusion, resulting in a lack of cellular oxygenation, multiple organ dysfunction, and death.

Cardiogenic Shock

Cardiogenic shock is most commonly caused by myocardial infarction. The development of shock depends on the amount of muscle wall damage that results from this insult. Other types of shock causing an inadequate circulation of blood may also lead to cardiogenic shock. When other types of shock are responsible, a myocardial depressant factor is released, which causes a severe depression of the heart muscle's ability to contract, resulting in a dilation of the left ventricle and leading to an inability of the heart to eject a sufficient amount of blood into the circulation.

Cardiogenic Shock Treatment

An intra–aortic balloon pump is most likely needed to assist the heart in propelling blood through the aorta. Fluid volume walks a tight rope between too much and too little. Hemodynamic monitoring is essential to regulate the IV fluids given to the patient. Enough fluid must be administered to keep the preload (ventricular filling pressure) sufficient and yet not too much to overburden an already taxed system. Correction of dysrhythmias and the use of inotropic agents (e.g., dopamine) may be necessary for maintaining blood pressure; however, decreasing the workload of the heart by decreasing afterload (systemic vascular resistance [SVR]) through vasodilators (e.g., nitroglycerine) is also important.

Circulatory Shock

A loss of circulating blood volume, whether actual or shifted among the fluid compartments, is the cause for circulatory shock. The end result is a lack of cellular oxygenation and eventual tissue and organ failure. Two types of circulatory shock are hypovolemic shock and obstructive shock.

Hypovolemic Shock

Hypovolemic shock occurs when approximately 15% to 20% of the blood volume is lost. It may occur with trauma resulting in hemorrhaging and a loss of whole blood, burns and a loss of plasma, or a loss of ECF such as with the GI system fluid loss through vomiting or diarrhea. Third spacing (i.e., the shifting of fluid from the vascular compartment to the interstitial or intracellular) or internal hemorrhaging also may cause hypovolemic shock.

Inadequate perfusion—the ultimate outcome of hypovolemic shock—starts with a decreased blood return to the heart, resulting in decreased cardiac output and circulatory insufficiency. The compensatory mechanisms of SNS stimulation, renin–angiotensin activation, and ADH stimulation will attempt to maintain the blood pressure and cardiac output.

Hypovolemic Shock Treatment

Treatment involves rapid fluid replacement. Surgical intervention may be needed if the insult is related to trauma. Success is achieved when blood pressure and cardiac output return to normal. A urine output of approximately 30 cc/hr indicates fluid balance has been achieved.

Obstructive Shock

Obstructive shock is related to some type of mechanical obstruction that interrupts blood flow through the circulation, heart, or lungs. Situations involving dissecting aortic aneurysm, cardiac tamponade, or pulmonary embolism are some of the more common factors causing obstructive shock. The obstruction of blood flow causes the pressures of the right side of the heart to elevate and impairs the return of blood to the heart, resulting in jugular vein distention and an elevated central venous pressure.

Obstructive Shock Treatment

Treatment includes correcting the problem and returning blood flow to normal. Maintaining blood pressure and cardiac output during this type of shock is difficult because blood flow is obstructed. Thrombolytics may work with pulmonary embolism, though multiple contraindications such as age, CPR, recent surgery, and others may prevent use of this therapy. Surgical repair of an aneurysm or removing fluid from the pericardial sac with tamponade may help to alleviate the blockage.

Distributive Shock

Distributive shock occurs because of an increased vascular compartment related to loss of blood vessel tone. The blood volume then becomes redistributed and a decreased volume is returned to the heart. This accounts for a decreased cardiac output and blood pressure. The important point to remember in distributive shock is that the blood volume is not diminished but redistributed. Three types of distributive shock exist: neurogenic shock, anaphylactic shock, and septic shock.

Neurogenic Shock

Neurogenic shock occurs secondary to a loss of vasomotor tone, which brings about vasodilation. Neurogenic shock may be caused by brain or spinal cord injury from a diving or bullet injury, lack of glucose to the brain, overdose of drugs, or anesthesia. In neurogenic shock, the skin is warm and dry. Cervical spinal cord injuries at or above the fifth thoracic vertebra result in the loss of SNS vasoconstrictor tone, causing an uncompensated massive vasodilation. In addition, hypotension occurs due to an unopposed parasympathetic nervous system action allowing for bradycardia, unlike other shock states in which tachycardia is a compensatory mechanism. Often the patient with spinal injury has hypothalamic dysfunction, causing a temperature dysfunction called *poikilothermy* (i.e., temperature of the environment). When combined with the vasodilation, the patient's temperature becomes even cooler.

Neurogenic Shock Treatment

Neurogenic shock is rare. If the cause is known, the condition may be corrected (e.g., neurogenic shock related to anesthesia can be reversed). Temporary administration of vasoconstrictors such as dopamine may be indicated. An insulin reaction causing decreased glucose availability for the brain can also be easily reversed through administration of glucose. Spinal cord injury is permanent and treatment of the shock state is comprehensive. Neurogenic shock related to spinal cord injury can develop immediately following the injury and last for days to weeks. Treatment involves fluid resuscitation and vasopressors, such as dopamine, to maintain cardiac output and tissue perfusion; phenylephrine or norepinephrine to increase the SVR; and management of the hypothermia with heating blankets.

Anaphylactic Shock

Anaphylaxis occurs when vasodilators such as histamine are released into the circulation as a result of an allergic reaction to drugs, foods, insect stings, or antitoxins.

The release of vasoactive mediators causes the vasodilation of arterioles and venules and makes the capillary wall permeable, which results in the leaking of fluid from the vascular to the interstitial space.

Initially, respiratory problems such as coughing, wheezing, and difficulty breathing occur. Bronchospasm and laryngeal edema develop, causing serious airway obstruction. Depending on the cause, itching and swelling of the lips, tongue, and eyes may occur. As with all distributive shock, the blood vessels dilate and the blood pools in the periphery, causing decreased blood pressure and cardiac output.

Anaphylactic Shock Treatment

Treatment includes prompt intervention with maintaining an open airway and oxygenation. Removing the cause is difficult since the insect bite or ingestion of substance has already occurred. Epinephrine or other antihistamines are essential for constricting blood vessels, smooth muscle relaxation to assist bronchodilation, and blockage of histamines.

Septic Shock

Septic shock is one of the most prevalent types of shock affecting hospitalized patients, though it can occur with healthy individuals who contract microorganisms that enter the bloodstream. As one of the most common types of distributive shock, it has a mortality rate of 50%. Hospitalized patients are most susceptible due to the use of invasive technology allowing for a portal of entry for the microorganism, coupled with an already immunocompromised system. The elderly are particularly susceptible due to a compromised immune system secondary to age and chronic diseases. In addition, if they are undergoing chemotherapy, their immune system becomes compromised from the drugs, making them vulnerable to microorganisms and potential sepsis.

Septic shock stems from an infection caused primarily by gram–negative bacteria; however, gram–positive bacteria, such as *Staphylococcus aureus* (responsible for toxic shock), can also be responsible. Regardless of the type of bacteria, the microorganism triggers components that release a cascade of events. Several theories exist attempting to explain the body's reaction to the microorganism. One theory speaks to toxins released from the microorganism that cause an immune reaction responsible for decreased vascular tone and increased permeability of the vascular system. This allows for a decreased SVR and vasodilation, which contributes to a maldistribution of the circulating blood volume and the hypotension that accompanies shock states. Another theory refers to systems such as complement, kinin, and the clotting cascade, which once released, cause widespread complications such as an increased permeability of the capillary wall and the development of the clotting syndrome, disseminated intravascular coagulation (DIC).

The clinical presentation of septic shock varies somewhat from the other types of shock. In the initial stages of septic shock, the patient looks uncompromised and may appear this way for hours to days prior to the start of the next stage. The skin is warm and dry with a rosy appearance due to the start of a decreased SVR and vasodilation. Personality changes and irritability may be present due to decreased cerebral blood flow. Respiratory alkalosis may also be present due to a slight hyperventilation. Urine output may be up to 100 cc/hr. Typically, the patient has a fever. The presentation of the patient in the initial stages of septic shock is that of a hyperdynamic state with a higher than normal cardiac output (compensatory mechanism for the decreased SVR) and normal to slightly decreased blood pressure and increased heart rate. However, if the shock progresses, increased vasodilation contributes to a lower blood pressure and the heart becomes dilated, unable to eject the necessary amount of blood required for adequate tissue perfusion.

Septic Shock Treatment

Treatment consists of identifying the source of infection and administering broad–spectrum and aminoglycoside antibiotics. Rapid infusion of IV fluids and vasopressor drugs to help increase the SVR are of importance. Hemodynamic monitoring of fluid balance is absolutely essential.

Fluid, Electrolyte, and Acid/Base Imbalance in Shock States

The fluid and electrolyte imbalances that occur with shock are vast. The BUN and creatinine elevate due to hypoperfusion and vasoconstriction of the renal system. Sodium increases during the early stages secondary to the increased secretion of aldosterone, but potassium decreases with renal excretion. Potassium increases as shock progresses due to the exchange with H^+ ions in acidosis and the release of potassium with cellular death. Calcium also increases in an acidotic state.

Acid/base balance swings from an alkalotic state to one of acidosis as the stages of shock progress. A respiratory alkalosis occurs during the beginning stages due to hyperventilation. Metabolic acidosis quickly ensues, however, with the accumulation of lactic acid from anaerobic metabolism.

Nursing Implications of Shock States

As mentioned throughout this chapter, different types of shock states involve varied medical treatment. Regardless of the type of shock, however, there are basic nursing assessments and interventions that are appropriate.

Neurologic checks and evaluation of the patient's level of consciousness are important indicators of cerebral blood flow. Behavioral manifestations of restlessness, irritability, confusion, and paresthesias are indicators of decreased cerebral blood flow. In addition to performing a neurologic assessment every hour, recording and reporting abnormal deviations and protecting the patient from injury are essential interventions.

Airway is of primary importance particularly with anaphylactic shock, but also with other shock–like states. Assessment of an increased/decreased rate, shallow or increased depth, use of accessory muscles or adventitious breath sounds, cyanosis, or dyspnea are indicators of respiratory distress. Administration of oxygen and ventilatory assistance may be required. Pulse oximetry to evaluate oxygen saturation and arterial blood gases for acid/base balance should be monitored. The lactic acidosis that develops with shock states does not require treatment with sodium bicarbonate unless the pH falls below 7.2. Generally, supplementary oxygen will help to increase tissue perfusion and fluid replacement will help to correct the acidotic state.

Assessment of vital signs, pulmonary artery pressures (PAP), pulmonary artery wedge pressures (PAWP), and cardiac output is necessary every 15 minutes if needed (PAWP is not taken as frequently due to complications with balloon rupture) and every hour as the patient stabilizes. Low blood pressure, postural hypotension, tachycardia or weak thready pulse, low PAP, and decreased urinary output are all indicators of fluid imbalance. Inotropic agents such as dopamine need to be titrated to support blood pressure. Cardiac monitoring is essential to prevent lethal dysrhythmias from developing secondary to electrolyte, acid/base, and fluid imbalance.

With the exception of cardiogenic shock, fluids such as normal saline are essential for volume expansion. Increased amounts of crystalloids are required because much of the volume will diffuse out of the vascular space secondary to increased capillary permeability and decreased oncotic pressure. Crystalloids, as large molecules, will be unable to leave the intravascular space and, in addition, will attract fluid helping to expand the intravascular compartment. Intake and output should be carefully measured on an hourly basis.

Monitoring signs and symptoms of overload through PAWP and urine output is important for evaluating renal function and to help assess fluid balance and adequate replacement. Measure urine output every hour. Assess and report laboratory values of elevated serum BUN and creatinine, low urine sodium, or blood in urine, which are all indicators of inadequate renal function.

Assessing for the presence of bowel sounds, distension, or abdominal pain should be conducted every 4 hours. Report problems of nausea and vomiting or diarrhea, which are all potential contributors to acid/base and electrolyte imbalances. Enteral feedings should be started as soon as the patient can tolerate them in order to meet metabolic demands.

Assess for peripheral vascular ischemia. Palpate all peripheral pulses and document and report complaints of pain, tingling, or numbness in the extremities. Evaluate the skin for pale or cyanotic color and for temperature as well as dryness. Helping the patient maintain a normal temperature is helpful for maintaining comfort and prevention of vasoconstriction. Proper skin care to maintain skin integrity is also important when the patient is immobile.

Fear and anxiety are concerns of the patient when aware of the severity of the situation. Assessing for sleeplessness, lack of communication, restlessness, or an increase in vital signs may indicate anxiety or a fear of death. Acknowledging the patient's feelings and showing concern are helpful for calming the patient and reducing anxiety.

PART V: QUESTIONS

1. What is the most common cause of acute renal failure?

(A) Hypertension

(B) Nephrotoxic injury

(C) Calculi

(D) ATN

2. Which of the following would be an example of a pre–renal factor that may cause acute renal failure?

(A) Clamping the aorta for more than 30 minutes during surgery

(B) Radiocontrast dyes

(C) Prostatic hyperplasia

(D) Renal tumor

3. Hyperkalemia in CRF results from _____ and _____.

(A) Oliguria/acidosis

(B) Increased urine output/low calcium levels

(C) Increased phosphate levels/low calcium levels

(D) Increased urine output/increased magnesium levels

4. Low levels of calcium occur in CRF due to:

(A) A decreased production of erythropoietin

(B) Elevated levels of phosphate

(C) Lack of vitamin D normally created by the kidneys

(D) An osmotic diuresis related to sodium loss

5. What is a V/Q mismatch?

(A) An anatomical shunt

(B) A V/Q discrepancy

(C) Decreased oxygen levels and increased alveolar CO_2 levels

(D) An inability to expel CO_2

6. Which of the following is a sign of right–sided heart failure?

(A) Blood backing up into the pulmonary bed

(B) Elevated PAWP

(C) Jugular venous distension and peripheral edema

(D) Decreased urine output

7. Which of the following is a hallmark sign of DKA?

(A) Hypertension

(B) Too much insulin

(C) Too few ketones

(D) Fruity breath

8. From which of the following does dehydration from HHNK result?

(A) Lack of insulin

(B) Elevated glucose levels

(C) Excess ketones

(D) Acidosis

9. Which of the following would indicate a deep partial–thickness burn injury?

(A) Mottled, waxy appearance

(B) Red, shiny, wet appearance

(C) Charred and dry skin

(D) Erythema and intact skin

10. Which stage of shock is the easiest stage to reverse the chain of events that lead to serious complications?

(A) Progressive

(B) Refractory

(C) Compensatory

(D) MODS

11. Which type of shock is a redistribution of blood not a loss of volume?

(A) Hypovolemic

(B) Distributive

(C) Cardiogenic

(D) Obstructive

12. The patient has a rosy appearance and the skin is warm and dry during the beginning phases of septic shock due to:

(A) Vasoconstriction

(B) Hypertension

(C) Increased vascular tone

(D) Vasodilation

1. The correct answer is D.

The most common cause of acute renal failure is ATN. Hypertension, injury caused by medications, and calculi do take their toll on the kidney but are not the most common cause.

2. The correct answer is A.

A prerenal cause for acute renal failure takes place outside of the renal system, causing a decreased blood flow to the kidneys. If blood flow is restored in time, damage to the kidneys is minimal. Radiocontrast dyes are an example of an intrarenal factor causing damage to the renal tissue/nephrons of the kidneys. Prostatic hyperplasia and renal tumor are examples of postrenal factors that cause an obstruction to the urologic structures.

3. The correct answer is A.

Potassium is eliminated in the urine and when little urine output exists, potassium accumulates. Also, during acidosis, the H+ ion moves into the cell in exchange for the potassium ion, contributing to the state of hyperkalemia. An increased urine output does not exist in CRF and the levels of calcium, magnesium, and phosphate are affected but do not contribute to hyperkalemia.

4. The correct answer is C.

The kidneys need to activate vitamin D in order for the GI system to absorb calcium. Because the kidneys lose that function in CRF, calcium is not absorbed and hypocalcemia results. The low calcium triggers the release of parathyroid hormone, which also releases phosphate, contributing to the high phosphate levels. Erythropoietin is a hormone produced by the kidneys that affects the RBC. Low calcium levels are not related to an osmotic diuresis.

5. The correct answer is B.

Ventilation and perfusion should be close to a 1:1 ratio. In certain respiratory conditions, ventilation may be affected and in others perfusion may be blocked, leading to a V/Q mismatch. An anatomical shunt occurs when blood enters the left side of the heart without passing through the lungs. Decreased oxygen levels and increased alveolar CO_2 refer to alveolar hypoventilation. An inability to expel CO_2 refers to hypercapnic respiratory failure.

6. The correct answer is C.

Jugular venous distention and peripheral edema are signs of blood backing up in the peripheral or systemic circulation from a failing right ventricle. Answers A and B are related to left–sided failure, though they eventually can be the cause of right–sided failure. A decreased urine output is not a sign of CHF; it may be associated with another disease process such as CRF in conjunction with CHF.

7. The correct answer is D.

The fruity breath is related to the excess ketones in the body and the breath takes on the smell of apple seeds (acetone). The condition results from too little insulin in relation to increased caloric intake or stress. Hypotension is common, not hypertension. Hypotension develops along with a weak rapid pulse due to low volume secondary to increased urine output.

8. The correct answer is B.

The elevated glucose causes an osmotic diuresis that leads to dehydration. The condition occurs with patients who are capable of producing insulin but not enough to counteract excess glucose. The main difference between DKA and HHNK is the lack of ketones and acidosis, as is present with HHNK.

9. The correct answer is A.

The second–degree deep partial–thickness injury takes on a mottled, waxy–white, or pink color with thin paper–like blisters. Answer B is a second–degree superficial partial–thickness burn. These injuries have skin that appears moist and weepy with blisters. Answer C is a fourth–degree burn and answer D is a first–degree burn.

10. The correct answer is C.

The compensatory stage is the initial stage when the body's compensatory mechanisms are attempting to keep up with the evolving process. Interceding at this stage is easiest since changes in VS, urine output, etc. are still subtle. The progressive stage begins to show a decrease in cardiac output, blood pressure, and an accumulation of acid. The refractory stage is virtually irreversible. MODS is the abbreviation for multiple organ dysfunction.

11. The correct answer is B.

Distributive shock occurs because the vascular compartment size has increased (i.e., lost tone redistributing the blood volume). Hypovolemic shock is an actual loss of blood volume. Cardiogenic shock is related to the inability of the heart to effectively pump blood to the tissues. Obstructive shock is related to a mechanical obstruction interrupting blood flow.

12. The correct answer is D.

The skin is warm and dry with a rosy appearance due to vasodilation. The vasodilation occurs due to a decreased vascular tone, allowing for more blood to pool into the peripheral areas and away from the major organs. Vasoconstriction leads to cool clammy skin because the blood is shunted away from the periphery. Hypertension does not occur in shock.

REFERENCES

Part I

Bullock, B., & Henze, R. (2000). *Focus on pathophysiology.* Philadelphia: Lippincott.

Copstead, L. E., & Banasik, J. (2000). *Pathophysiology biological and behavioral perspectives* (2nd ed.). Philadelphia: Saunders.

Huether, S., & McCance, K. (2000). *Understanding pathophysiology* (2nd ed.). St. Louis, MO: Mosby.

Kaplan, J. (2002). Biochemistry of Na, K–ATPase. *Annual Review of Biochemistry, 71,* 511–535.

Kee, J., & Paulanka, B. (2000). *Handbook of fluid, electrolyte and acid–base imbalances.* Albany, NY: Delmar.

Lewis, S., Heitkemper, M., Dirkesen, S., O'Brien, P., Giddens, J., & Bucher, L. (2004). *Medical–surgical nursing assessment and management of clinical problems* (6th ed.). St. Louis, MO: Mosby.

Porth, C. (2002). *Pathophysiology concepts of altered health states* (6th ed.). Philadelphia: Lippincott.

Price, S., & Wilson, L. (2003). *Pathophysiology clinical concepts of disease processes* (6th ed.). St. Louis, MO: Mosby.

Part II

Beck, L. (2000). The aging kidney: Defending a delicate balance of fluid and electrolytes. *Geriatrics, 55*(4), 26–32.

Bigard, A. X., Sanchez, H., & Claveyrolas, G. (2001). Effects of dehydration and rehydration on EMG changes during fatiguing contractions. *Medicine and Science in Sports and Exercise, 33*(10), 1694–1700.

Bullock, B., & Henze, R. (2000). *Focus on pathophysiology.* Philadelphia: Lippincott.

Castiglione, V. (2000). Emergency hyperkalemia. *American Journal of Nursing, 100*(1), 55–56.

Copstead, L. E., & Banasik, J. (2000). *Pathophysiology biological and behavioral perspectives* (2nd ed.). Philadelphia: Saunders.

Gisolfi, C., Lambert, P., & Summers, R. (2001). Intestinal fluid absorption during exercise: Role of sport drink osmolality and (Na+). *Medicine and Science in Sports and Exercise, 33*(6), 907–915.

Halperin, M., & Kamel, K. (1998). Potassium. *Lancet, 52*(9122), 135–149.

Huether, S., & McCance, K. (2000). *Understanding pathophysiology* (2nd ed.). St. Louis, MO: Mosby.

Kee, J., & Paulanka, B. (2000). *Handbook of fluid, electrolyte and acid–base imbalances.* Albany, NY: Delmar.

Lewis, S., Heitkemper, M., Dirkesen, S., O'Brien, P., Giddens, J., & Bucher, L. (2004). *Medical–surgical nursing assessment and management of clinical problems* (6th ed.). St. Louis, MO: Mosby.

Mao, I. F., Chen, M. L., & Ko, Y. C. (2001). Electrolyte loss in sweat and iodine deficiency in a hot environment. *Archives of Environmental Health, 56*(3), 271–277.

Messinger–Rapport, B., & Thacker, H. (2002). Prevention for older woman: A practical guide to prevention and treatment of osteoporosis. *Geriatrics, 57*(4), 16–27.

Miller, M. (1998). Hyponatremia: Age–related risk factors and therapy decisions. *Geriatrics, 53*(7), 32–43.

Porth, C. (2002). *Pathophysiology concepts of altered health states* (6th ed.). Philadelphia: Lippincott.

Price, S., & Wilson, L. (2003). *Pathophysiology clinical concepts of disease processes* (6th ed.). St. Louis, MO: Mosby.

Sabatini, B. L., & Regehr, W. G. (1999). Timing of synaptic transmission. *Annual Review of Physiology, 61,* 521–542.

Schmidt, W., Rojas, J., & Boning, D. (1999). Plasma–electrolytes in natives to hypoxia after marathon races at different altitudes. *Medicine and Science in Sports and Exercise, 31*(10), 1406–1413.

The minerals we need. (2003). *Harvard Women's Health Watch, 10*(9), 5–6.

Weiss, M., & Sankaran, G. (1998). A health education initiative: Teaching college women about osteoporosis. *Journal of Nursing Education, 37*(6), 271–274.

Wexler, R. (2002). Evaluation and treatment of heat–related illnesses. *American Family Physician, 65*(11), 2307–2314.

Part III

Bullock, B., & Henze, R. (2000). *Focus on pathophysiology.* Philadelphia: Lippincott.

Copstead, L. E., & Banasik, J. (2000). *Pathophysiology biological and behavioral perspectives* (2nd ed.). Philadelphia: Saunders.

Huether, S., & McCance, K. (2000). *Understanding pathophysiology* (2nd ed.). St. Louis, MO: Mosby.

Kaplan, J. (2002). Biochemistry of Na, K–ATPase. *Annual Review of Biochemistry, 71,* 511–535.

Kee, J., & Paulanka, B. (2000). *Handbook of fluid, electrolyte and acid–base imbalances.* Albany, NY: Delmar.

Lewis, S., Heitkemper, M., Dirkesen, S., O'Brien, P., Giddens, J., & Bucher, L. (2004). *Medical–surgical nursing assessment and management of clinical problems* (6th ed.). St. Louis, MO: Mosby.

Porth, C. (2002). *Pathophysiology concepts of altered health states* (6th ed.). Philadelphia: Lippincott.

Price, S., & Wilson, L. (2003). *Pathophysiology clinical concepts of disease processes* (6th ed.). St. Louis, MO: Mosby.

Stephens, T., McKenna, M., & Canny, B. (2002). Effect of sodium bicarbonate on muscle metabolism during intense endurance cycling. *Medicine and Science in Sports and Exercise, 34*(4), 614–621.

Part IV

Bullock, B., & Henze, R. (2000). *Focus on pathophysiology.* Philadelphia: Lippincott.

Copstead, L. E., & Banasik, J. (2000). *Pathophysiology biological and behavioral perspectives* (2nd ed.). Philadelphia: Saunders.

Huether, S., & McCance, K. (2000). *Understanding pathophysiology* (2nd ed.). St. Louis, MO: Mosby.

Kaplan, J. (2002). Biochemistry of Na, K–ATPase. *Annual Review of Biochemistry, 71*, 511–535.

Kee, J., & Paulanka, B. (2000). *Handbook of fluid, electrolyte and acid–base imbalances.* Albany, NY: Delmar.

Lewis, S., Heitkemper, M., Dirkesen, S., O'Brien, P., Giddens, J., & Bucher, L. (2004). *Medical–surgical nursing assessment and management of clinical problems* (6th ed.). St. Louis, MO: Mosby.

Porth, C. (2002). *Pathophysiology concepts of altered health states* (6th ed.). Philadelphia: Lippincott.

Price, S., & Wilson, L. (2003). *Pathophysiology clinical concepts of disease processes* (6th ed.). St. Louis, MO: Mosby.

Part V

Ammon, S. (2001). Managing patients with heart failure. *American Journal of Nursing, 101*(12), 26–33.

Beck, L. (2000). The aging kidney: Defending a delicate balance of fluid and electrolytes. *Geriatrics, 55*(4), 26–32.

Bullock, B., & Henze, R. (2000). *Focus on pathophysiology.* Philadelphia: Lippincott.

Carelock, J., & Clark, A. (2001). Heart failure: Pathophysiologic mechanisms. *American Journal of Nursing, 101*(12), 26–33.

Copstead, L. E., & Banasik, J. (2000). *Pathophysiology biological and behavioral perspectives* (2nd ed.). Philadelphia: Saunders.

Futterman, L., & Lemberg, L. (2003). Diuretics, the most critical therapy in heart failure, yet often neglected in the literature. *American Journal of Critical Care, 121*(4), 376–380.

Huether, S., & McCance, K. (2000). *Understanding pathophysiology* (2nd ed.). St. Louis, MO: Mosby.

Kaplan, J. (2002). Biochemistry of Na, K–ATPase. *Annual Review of Biochemistry, 71*, 511–535.

Kee, J., & Paulanka, B. (2000). *Handbook of fluid, electrolyte and acid–base imbalances.* Albany, NY: Delmar.

Lewis, S., Heitkemper, M., Dirkesen, S., O'Brien, P., Giddens, J., & Bucher, L. (2004). *Medical–surgical nursing assessment and management of clinical problems* (6th ed.). St. Louis, MO: Mosby.

Mann, H., & Stiller, S. (2000). Sodium modeling. *Kidney International Supplement, 76*, 79–88.

Marks, J. B. (2003). Perioperative management of diabetes. *American Family Physician, 67*(1), 93–100.

Miller, M. (1998). Hyponatremia: Age–related risk factors and therapy decisions. *Geriatrics, 53*(7), 32–43.

Porth, C. (2002). *Pathophysiology concepts of altered health states* (6th ed.). Philadelphia: Lippincott.

Price, S., & Wilson, L. (2003). *Pathophysiology clinical concepts of disease processes* (6th ed.). St. Louis, MO: Mosby:.

Stefanidis, I., Stiller, S., Ikonomov, V., & Mann, H. (2002). Sodium and body fluid homeostasis in profiling hemodialysis treatment. *The International Journal of Artificial Organs, 25*(5), 421–428.

INDEX